Confessions of a Medicine Man

D1176914

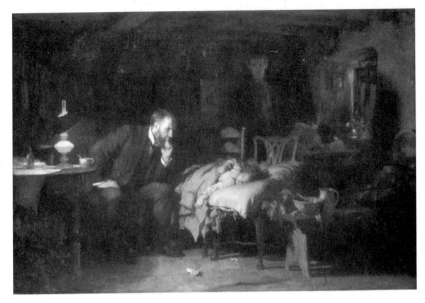

Sir Luke Fildes. *The Doctor, 1891*. Tate Gallery, London/Art Resource, New York

Confessions of a Medicine Man
An Essay in Popular Philosophy

Alfred I. Tauber

A Bradford Book
The MIT Press
Cambridge, Massachusetts
London, England

First MIT Press paperback edition, 2000
© 1999 Massachusetts Institute of Technology

This book was set in Sabon by Crane Composition, Inc. and was printed and bound in the United States of America.

Library of Congress Cataloging-in-Publication Data

Tauber, Alfred I.
  Confessions of a medicine man : an essay in popular philosophy / Alfred I. Tauber.
    p.   cm.
  "A Bradford book."
  Includes bibliographical references and index.
  ISBN 0-262-20114-3 (hardcover : alk. paper), 0-262-70072-7 (pb)
  1. Medical ethics. 2. Medicine—Philosophy. 3. Physician and patient—Moral and ethical aspects. I. Title.
R724.T38   1998
174'.2—dc21   98-27288
                                                          CIP

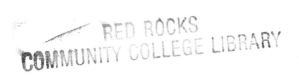

For Paula

Contents

Acknowledgments

Confessions of a Medicine Man seems to me like an aged cheese or bottle of wine. Begun in 1992 and put away for another five years, this essay has actually cured for decades, indeed my whole life, from earliest childhood to adulthood. The book began innocently enough as a series of anecdotes from my clinical medical practice, but soon became an autobiographical exploration of professional life, in which I have commented on my career as a physician from the perspective of philosophy. More than an opportunity for recollection, reminiscence, and reflection, in many ways this narrative refashions and synthesizes the corpus of my work over the past decade in the history and philosophy of science and medicine. Whether writing on the nineteenth-century origins of immunology, the scientific philosophy of Goethe, or the nature of reductive thinking in biology, I now see that my entire research effort has been informed and guided by a particular moral understanding. At the most obvious level, my formal scholarly efforts have attempted to erect conceptual bridges between the domains of the clinic and laboratory on the one hand and philosophy on the other. Key to that effort was my endeavor to ally seemingly disparate worldviews under a common humane banner.

My colleagues on both sides of the divide have supported this effort with uncommon generosity, and I deeply appreciate having been able to play an active role in both worlds. To engage undergraduates and graduate students in the philosophical questions that intrigue me, as well as to continue practicing hematology, calls upon very different kinds of intellectual endeavor. Their integration, the constant interplay of philosophical reflection on medicine and the practical concerns of the world on philosophy, serves as the diverse source stimulating my professional and intellectual life. For me, the institutional flexibility that has allowed these pursuits reflects academic freedom, inasmuch as I followed interests that would not neatly fall into one department or another. In the world of academia, institutional boundaries are usually patrolled borders. The Departments of Medicine and Pathology at the Boston University School of Medicine and the Department of Philosophy at Boston University suffer no such xenophobia, and I salute my humanistic colleagues who have made me, initially a stranger, welcome. I cannot imagine having written this book in another environment.

The issues discussed, the arguments made, the conclusions drawn, reflect many informal and academic discussions with friends and colleagues too numerous to name or formally acknowledge. But several have read drafts of the manuscript and helped me clarify the narrative. Of special note are Richard Adler, George Annas, Robert S. Cohen, Anne Dubitzsky, Shimon Glick, Scott Podolsky, David Roochnik, and Roger Shattuck. To them, I can only offer special thanks for supporting my efforts and helping me bring forth the book I have yearned to write for a very long time.

I am also indebted to the staff at The MIT Press, especially Betty Stanton for her enthusiastic support and Judy Feldmann for her keen editorial judgment. An integration of my various personae, professional and personal, this essay truly is a "confession," an attempt to draw upon my most intimate experiences as a resource for our common moral understanding. To all those who have helped me clarify the issues that focus this inquiry, I give heartfelt thanks. Finally, I navigated my way in this book through a complex personal triangulation, and although the bearings are, of course, my own, I was steadied by Paula Fredriksen, to whom this book is dedicated with my deepest admiration and love.

A. I. T.
Boscawen, NH
August, 1997

Introduction

Sometimes, not too often, I can't sleep. I lie in bed, turning from one side to another, my mind tossing on a sea of feelings, ideas, events, problems, angers, fears. Last night, somewhere between midnight and early dawn, I remembered Tony DiVilo. He was six years old in the spring of 1976 and I was still training to become a hematologist. Tony had leukemia, and for six months he had been resistant to chemotherapy. There was no bone marrow donor match. Tony was about the same age as my first son. They both had wiry, active bodies, bright eyes, and coy grins. Tony however hardly ever smiled when his father brought him to the clinic. His mother never came (she never did) and I never met her. There were four other siblings. I never saw them either. Only Tony and his father.

One morning, I remember it was a bright day, I took a call from Mr. DiVilo. Tony was very drowsy, could not be roused. I said to bring the child immediately to the hospital. They took a cab.

Mr. DiVilo walked into the waiting room carrying Tony, draped in his arms exactly like Michelangelo's Pieta. *The body was grey, and serenely beautiful. A black lock of hair over his forehead. The eyes closed. The father handed me his child, whom I took to an examining room and placed on a table. I was alone with him, and waves of emotion charged through me as I peered at his lifeless body. I was numb. I did not cry. I did not go to the funeral. I never spoke with Mr. DiVilo again. I ran away.*

Lying in bed, thinking of Tony, and then others, I resolved to write my confessions. I then fell into deep sleep.

I began my medical career in a different era, not so much as measured in years, but a seemingly distant, nostalgic past when viewed from our current vantage. It was, at least in this domain, a more innocent period, when patients went to doctors and expected a kind of care that has increasingly become difficult to find even if one has strong financial resources. I am referring to a time when the doctor's relationship with his or her patient was sacrosanct.

Not long ago, medical decisions were almost always made on the basis of trust; economic and administrative restraints were minimized; fears of malpractice were faint. Patients respected their physicians, the public had the highest esteem for the medical profession, and the physician was rarely the employee of anyone. The idea of a forty-hour work week for a doctor was to relegate him to a regular profession, ruled by everyday standards. A plumber might show up a day late or not at all; the physician was accountable to another principle, and with good reason. A backed-up toilet was a problem; illness or the threat of death was a calamity.

The family doctor is now legend, not only because the physician has increasingly become part of a corporate operation, which by its very character is a process machine, but also because of a shift in the doctor-patient relationship. This essay explores that interpersonal tie, the fundamental unit in medicine. To examine the basis of the ethic governing the caregiver is to understand the very foundation of what it is to be ill and the role of the physician or nurse in helping to restore health. I am concerned with nothing less than the ethical commitment to make each of us whole when diseased.

Perhaps the best snapshot of today's medicine is the TV commercial or newspaper advertisement depicting a smiling nurse or doctor looking with apparent compassion at either a child or an elderly patient. Why? First, the doctor-patient relationship is primary. Just as beer commercials feature beer bottles, and car commercials feature cars, health care advertisements show the profession's essential relationship. Medicine is caring. But there is a second, perhaps more subtle reason the media attempts to capture an ostensibly normal scene of compassion. I suspect that they recognize that the five-minute clinic visit, the cog-in-the-wheel attitude so rampant in today's health care facility, is the source of great anxiety. The commercial denies dehumanization, selling the product of heath care just as one might sell a vacation to Bermuda or a sneaker called Air Jordan. And of course we buy. We need affordable health care and we want to be reassured. Are we? The happy scene sold on television is obviously part of a complex marketing strategy intertwined with the economics of production. And we all know it.

The health-care industry is the largest in America, accounting for one in every seven dollars of the gross domestic product (GDP). Assuming about 5 percent of the GDP in 1960, by 1995 the share had dramatically risen to almost 14 percent. Because of the extraordinary inflation in the health care industry in the late 1970s and throughout the 1980s, where health care coverage for employees was rising as much as 20 percent a year, managed care became the *de facto* health policy of the United States. The revolution in provider care is clearly illustrated by the following statistic: In 1987, 95 percent of Americans who received health coverage through their employment received close to full repayment for medical services from physicians and hospitals of their own choosing. Today, half of them have lost that freedom and now receive their care from health maintenance organizations chosen by their employers. Decisions about cost savings and rationing of resources were alien to the health care provider twenty-five years ago, and as a physician I have found that my profession has increasingly added a new dimension to its professional profile: We have become patient advocates in the attempt to resist the often insidious, too often draconian measures taken by nameless administrators to make health care more efficient and profitable. They are not necessarily evil—they are simply governed by a different ethos.

Medicine has always been a business. It used to be a middle class operation; today it is big business, and methods developed for selling products like cereal have been adapted for processing the ill and selling health care. Moreover, profits formerly funneled back into hospitals and medical schools are now siphoned off as corporate dividends. When one compares commercial with nonprofit medical plans, a telling statistic emerges: A recent *Consumer Reports* study found that whereas the nonprofits spent over 90 percent of their revenues on their patients, the commercial entities spent 79 percent on health care, allocating the rest to advertising, investors, and dividends. For instance, in 1996 United Health Care paid a 16 percent return. That was $356 million! The business of caring for the sick is apparently highly profitable despite the reduction of health-care cost inflation.

In the quest to achieve maximum utility and efficiency of the health care budget, profit-seeking entities are realizing a large benefit. That problem will ultimately require a political solution. This is doubtless a critical issue, but it is not my province. I am a physician, not a health care manager, nor a politician. My interests concern serving the patient. Medicine is a calling based on a special social relationship. We see parallel demands made upon teachers and clergy, and thus medicine is not singular in requiring an ethos of caring. But the strains put upon doctors and nurses in respect to challenging that ethos seem to me unique. I offer this essay to address the ways in which the industrialization of medicine is supported by the way we think of each other. The economic and political agendas have changed, but in addition, the standards governing medical practice seem to be shifting. I believe that we may be subject to altered expectations in regard to medical care not only because we are realistically facing new challenges posed by the cost of health care to society at large, but also because the fundamental relationships governing the way we interact with each other are less civil and less cohesive than we might hope.

Each of us has been and will at sometime in the future be ill. At those times of vulnerability we seek and expect compassionate care. But our confidence that such care will be available is deteriorating. We see the signs everywhere, and we rail against the most egregious attempts to ration care: Proposals such as outpatient mastectomies and discharging women the day after childbirth result in headlines. They only reflect the growing anger that we have lost control of our medical care to insurers and corporate health centers, whose primary concerns are those of any corporation— profits, not patients. Despite reassurances that Mr. and Mrs. Joe Public are satisfied, I know, my colleagues know, and the public knows that something crucial to our sense of probity in this arena has gone awry.

"Willie Jones needs Panzola."
  "So?"
  "So, he has no insurance."
  "He's got Medicare."
  "Right. They won't pay for the drug."

"He can try for special reimbursement."

"First, they probably won't reimburse, and second, he doesn't have enough money to buy it up front."

"We can try to get the company to send it on compassion."

"I've had poor luck. When I applied last time they delayed so long and sent so little it was just about too late."

"What about the patient fund?"

"I've talked to Gail. She says there's no money left and we can't get a renewal for 60 days."

"Does the pharmacy have any extra bottles?"

"I called Herb; either they don't or he won't."

"So what are you going to do?"

"Either nothing, or admit him."

"The ward won't solve the problem. It'll buy him a week or two, then he'll be discharged. The blood will thicken and you're at ground zero."

"I'll buy time. Maybe something will turn up."

"Hmm . . ."

"The alternative is to do nothing."

"That's what I'd do. He's hit the brick wall before."

"Yeah, but this time will be his last."

This essay is written not in anger nor even in protest, but the sources of its concern reside in a response to the challenges we now face to preserve medicine's most fundamental charge: its commitment to the care of the patient. My mission is to analyze medicine's ethical structure. I do so as both a physician and a philosopher—and my voice in the second role is informed by my voice in the first. I have lived with the growing encumbrances that have imposed themselves on myself and my patients. As a philosopher I have sought to examine why we have had so little clarity on how to rectify our dissatisfaction; as a physician I have sought professional solutions to the frustrations of fighting a medical system that has become increasingly hostile to my standards of care for my patients. Here as both a philosopher and a doctor, I will explore the ethical issues I believe are the root of our predicament.

We require a critical reexamination—and a radical reorientation—of the ethos of medicine to correct what has gone wrong. To fortify if not recapture an ever-fading image of medical care, I present here my testimony. A loose narrative of my evolution as a physician weaves in and out of an essay in popular philosophy; the vignettes serve both to explain the evolution of my career as a doctor and to illustrate the ethical points discussed in the philosophical argument, which itself requires no technical expertise to comprehend.

The stories indeed form part of the philosophical discussion and should not be regarded as divorced from or even complementary to the more formal deliberations. Narrative itself formulates ethical problems and solutions. Novels, poems, plays, personal accounts—all offer vivid moral lessons not by elaborating a systematic ethics but by tapping into collective experience and the wellsprings of the "social imaginary." It is here that we encounter moral choice—solution and impasse—in the full panoply of human behavior. As contemporary philosopher Alasdair MacIntyre writes, "I can only answer the question 'What am I to do?' if I can answer the prior question 'Of what story or stories do I find myself a part?' " Narrative thus not only becomes a legitimate source for philosophical comment but presents us with the very possibility of developing moral inquiry.

The use of personal story to frame philosophical questions of moral knowledge is a tradition in Western letters stretching back at least as far as Augustine (354–430), whose own *Confessions*, through the appeal and power of his introspective narrative, still engage even the modern reader. Those *Confessions* stand stylistically as a triptych: the autobiographical illustration of his philosophical principles forms the first panel (Books 1–9); his contemplation of the moral, epistemological, and integrative life of memory, the second (Book 10); the direct application of these earlier insights to his immediate imperative—knowing God through Creation— the third (Books 11–13). His recount is so compelling and immediate, however, that too often the modern reader's interest ends with Book 9. We mistake his ingenious essay for "simple" autobiography, and so miss the specifically philosophical restatement of the questions by which he shaped his life story, and the answers he has to give. Surely the power of his personal narrative informs and enriches his more formal philosophy, which in itself is an interesting comment about the nature of his discourse. But the critical point to emphasize is that Augustine's *Confessions* are first and foremost not autobiography, but philosophy.

In this regard, my own memories are used as a narrative vehicle to present my philosophical position, and in part to minimize the chances of a similar misreading, I have followed a different strategy in presenting my own *Confessions*. If a triptych is the visual stylistic analogue to Augustine's, a Jackson Pollock painting perhaps best analogizes mine. Personal stories and distillations of my own professional experience, a short history of modern American medical practice, a quick march through Western moral philosophy—all these themes play and interweave throughout. Each serves, I hope, to enunciate the ethics I argue for here. Because the moral discourse emerges in my narrative, my vignettes are integral to the philosophical fabric of this essay.

Do not be daunted by *philosophy*. It need not be remote or arcane. To be sure, philosophy has become a complex discipline not easily accessible to the nonprofessional, but it clearly deserves a place in public discourse. Popular philosophy is not simple, but it should be available to help decipher problems from its own unique vantage and to offer solutions that are readily applicable to our world. American philosophy has a long tradition of contributing to public debate, and this essay takes its place in that tradition. Specifically, the historical developments in medicine have bequeathed us an identity problem, namely, what professional ideal we wish to instill and develop in our health care providers. The solution I am seeking rests on an analysis of the philosophical issues as a means of responding to this challenge. Here is an opportunity for philosophy to truly exhibit the power of its approach. Obviously, medical ethics may be examined from diverse perspectives arising from various cultural, historical, legal, and political frameworks. But philosophy isolates the conceptual question pertinent to moral agency within the domain of ethics itself, independent of other confounding and confusing elements. Although related to ethical issues, the other contexts in which medical ethics may be discussed bring to the table their own agendas, which while relevant must remain separate matters.

I intend this book not only for those who work in the health-care professions, but also for the general public, to alert both the ill and their advocates to how we might renew our efforts to make medicine more humane and compassionate. If we better understand the conceptual framework which guides our general sense of moral choice in the setting of warding off disease, then perhaps we will strengthen our efforts to establish an ethic of caring that is both passionate and scientific, care that truly is comprehensive to our human needs. This is a widely held goal, but in my discussions with physicians there seems to be an almost universal resignation to the power of economic and administrative forces to herd the clinician into a rigid and confined moral space. No doubt the challenge to resist has been heard, but our collective resolve seems to be wavering. Yet we must recognize that choices *do* loom before us and that those options must be clarified amidst the confusion of change. It has become a moral challenge to reassert the earliest calling of the medical profession. These confessions are offered as a response to that opportunity.

Confessions of a Medicine Man

1

Turmoil and Challenges

Utopia?

The intern was sharp. His white jacket and trousers were spotless and neatly pressed. His hair was carefully parted, not a misplaced strand. He wore a tie perfectly knotted and hanging at just the right length at the belt buckle. He was reciting the case history to Dr. Windsor and his retinue of students, residents, fellows, and nurses. Ten of us were huddled in the hall, listening attentively.

"The patient is a 67-year-old Caucasian female, whose chief complaint is upper abdominal pain. She was admitted last night with a twelve-hour history of unremitting pain and intermittent vomiting. . . ."

He intoned a detailed history, summarily reviewing pertinent past medical history and other relevant information, and then reciting the laboratory data, seemingly endless numbers. He had examined the blood smear himself and had performed the urinalysis. The entire monologue was given without benefit of notes and any reference to the chart. He knew his patient, and everyone in attendance knew that he knew.

It was the first time I had witnessed such a presentation. I was impressed. More, I was awed. Would I ever learn that much? How could he remember every detail? Did he make it up? Impossible. Dr. Windsor was perusing the chart; the senior medical resident was nodding in agreement. When the discussion of the case ensued, the intern moved from chronicler to commentator. With seeming ease he listed the differential diagnoses, a compendium of possible explanations, and then he proceeded to the plan for evaluation and finally therapy.

When he finished, Dr. Windsor looked up and said "Why didn't you get an abdominal echo? You might've missed a dissecting aortic aneurysm. Really . . . quite intolerable."

The intern was speechless and looked down. Appropriately humbled, he followed Dr. Windsor into the patient's room, where the professor initiated his own analysis with, "I've heard a bit about you, Mrs. Ford, but I need to ask you some more questions."

Twenty-five years ago medicine was approaching the cusp of what we now call "the health care crisis." As a medical student, I looked about and saw nothing but heady optimism. In retrospect, it was the Golden Age of American medicine. The turmoil of the 1960s seemed focused on race, sex, and war. Medicine was somehow above such concerns. We lived in the hospital. We took care of the ill. We responded to the needy. Society was racked with self-examination and radical criticism, but we were committed to science, the pure ethos of caring, and the advancement of our profession. We wore white and rode above the fray. Somehow, like Ernest Hemingway driving his ambulance in World War I Italy, I felt innocently immune to the travail with which society was reexamining its premises and priorities. I simply focused on becoming a doctor, and I was happy to follow the established course. And that prescription had been defined for over half a century as a scientific ethos.

The most respected professors were clinical investigators. Almost exclusively men, they had devoted their careers to the laboratory, seeking new diagnostic tests and novel therapeutic modalities. These doctors were the ones rewarded with professorships and the accolades of the profession. They reflected medicine's highest ideals, and I was awed by them. But unknown to any of us, their standing was tottering on the edge of a vast abyss of doubt. The values that had enshrined their endeavor were now open to question. These included the notion that progress in medicine—as in the science upon which it was based—knew no limits. This enthusiasm had many manifestations, but one that stood out for all to see was the general consent that costs were not of concern in the case of ministering to the ill. Whatever test was required, whatever surgical procedure might be deemed worthy of offering a chance at improving health or lengthening life, would be used without economic restraint. Insurance or government would pick up the costs and any consideration of expense simply was outside our interests. When the economic crisis of accounting finally began to ration health care delivery, we were all taken by surprise. After all, medicine was the sacred cow of American society.

But the refashioning of medicine had deeper roots than merely financial, and the assault, when finally declared, garnered power from diverse sources. Because medicine is so interwoven into the fabric of our culture, the early attack was disguised, and we hardly knew that a siege was on. However, in retrospect, we can now recognize that the triumphs of the medical-industrial complex in the middle of this century were subject to the same critical gaze that Americans were directing toward all major cultural institutions. Education, sexuality, race, and foreign policy were the most visible, but medicine was also under scrutiny. The cultural history of that period, roughly between the assassination of John Kennedy and the *de facto* impeachment of Richard Nixon, may retrospectively be regarded as a merciless dissecting and analyzing, in meticulous detail, of all of our assumptions regarding what we so lazily viewed as basic American values. And the debate introduced arguments heretofore unsounded. In short, a radical examination was under way, in which criteria recently hardly recognized as relevant were becoming regarded as cogent. Medicine would not escape similar inquiry, and the questions were about to expose the fragile balance between the clinical agendas of patient care and scientific knowledge.

The irony was that medicine seemed so insulated from criticism. If the infant mortality rate was too high in poverty-stricken areas, this was viewed as a reflection of economic and government policies. Medicare and Medicaid were enacted to help rectify such imbalances, and physicians were simply to serve as the agents, and beneficiaries, of the government. Similarly, in 1964 the Hill-Burton Act was passed to help communities build hospitals, and again this was viewed as the product of a new social awareness that equality of medical care was to be pursued. After all, wasn't medicine universally regarded as a noble cause, and moreover a huge success, and thus deserving of political and social investment? Clinical practice had followed a scientific agenda, which was perceived as paying huge dividends. The federal government was investing heavily in basic clinical research and the training of scientific medical specialists. The insurance companies—actually, Mr. and Mrs. Joe Public—were liberally reimbursing hospitals and physicians for new therapies and diagnostics, oblivious to costs. Physicians enjoyed the highest respect ratings of all professions, and they commensurately earned the highest incomes. Their social and economic status was about to receive a major trimming. This is not the place to explore why physicians were scrutinized and how they were demoted, but suffice it to note that a dissatisfaction took root that was articulated in diverse ways, none more pressing than the growing costs of health care. Americans took a careful look at their pocketbooks and concluded that they were not getting enough for their money. Broadly speaking, there were two major components to this dissatisfaction: resentment directed against the physician and an impatience with unmet expectations.

Despite indignant disavowals, the financial rewards of medicine were seen increasingly as corrupting. Conflicts of interest were exposed and unnecessary procedures and tests documented. Malpractice suits rose in number and monetary awards to the claimants increased dramatically, in part as a response to the avaricious practices of physicians, but also because the medical profession was generally being held to a more critical standard of conduct. During the reassessment of our major social institutions that followed in the wake of the tumult of the late 1960s, physicians suddenly were viewed with a jaundiced eye. In a fundamental sense they had lost their status as demigods. Such standing in previous generations had been based on personal sacrifice, uncommon intelligence or accomplishment, and the authority of scientific power. But each of these attributes was now subject to profound doubt. The physician was no longer of humble middle class, having become a wealthy entrepreneur; he potentially abused his trust, as evinced by the malpractice crisis. In addition, the public increasingly voiced disenchantment with the very scientific ethos of medicine. This disgruntlement takes many forms, and I will briefly sketch here only the economic issues that are pertinent to our use of technology, our support of basic research, and our assessment of benefits of standard clinical care.

One of today's most evident frustrations with medicine pertains to the clinician's growing reliance on technology, whose ascendancy is striking in both scope and character. One measure is simply to take an economic accounting. As David Rothman has documented in *Beginnings Count: The Technological Imperative in American Health Care*, per capita expenditures on medical instruments and supplies in the mid-1990s were almost eight times what they were in 1960. New drugs, diagnostic imaging, and surgical techniques account for much of what might be deemed progress, but there are less obviously necessary increased expenditures in disposable daily supplies, fancy thermometers, digital monitors, and the like. The cost/benefit ratio of new technologies is not at all clear in most cases, and we are still guided by the general ethic that life is precious and any expense is worthwhile in its preservation. So, although cost/benefit ratios are very high, close to a third of Medicare's budget is spent on the last year of patients' lives. The enormous cost of the newer technologies responsible for this expense has led to a growing suspicion that perhaps our health care dollars could be better spent. Even in the case of less dire choices regarding more routine medical options, we may not always be getting the best value with fancier whistles and bells. The true scandal is that we do not really know how efficient or appropriate is the use of most of our new technology. What may seem to be well-spent resources are often championed by parties interested in using them for either economic or professional self-aggrandizement.

In discussions of the medical industry, the public generally makes no distinction between science and its application, technology. Thus anger over rising health care costs has spilled over into a debate concerning the allocation of resources to various basic research programs that are hoped to lead to clinical innovations. Demands for more direct applications of laboratory science to new technologies is a radical departure from the independence, if not the sanctity, of basic research.

The promise of science, actually applied science in the form of new technologies, has been proclaimed as a panacea bringing health and longevity for over a century. With the discovery of infectious diseases at the end of the nineteenth century and the strategies of discovering "magic bullets" to eradicate microbial pathogens (the antisyphilis drug Salvarsan in 1907, sulfur in the 1930s, and penicillin in the 1940s), science declared a program of rational medicine that has served as the basis of modern diagnostics and therapeutics. The rationality of those claims has remained intact, and the results of antibiotics on the one hand, and eradication programs of insect vectors on the other, were dramatic chapters of science-based medicine. Despite the heady enthusiasm of that era, which lasted roughly from the mid-1870s into the 1950s, the results of a laboratory-based medicine have been increasingly scrutinized and the verdict has been more circumspect than earlier predictions.

There is no doubt that we have made notable progress in fighting certain diseases, but increasingly we appreciate that simple changes in sanitation, diet, and lifestyles (such as quitting smoking or exercising regularly) have had more dramatic effects on public health than more highly touted advances in conquering particular diseases. It is difficult to state in clear categorical terms the cost/benefit relationships for resources spent on basic research. The National Institutes of Health has in recent years endeavored to define more carefully our research goals in regard to targeted clinical ends, but the data that would allow an assessment of how scientific and technological achievements translate into a higher quality of health care or objective health criteria are difficult to obtain. Without this information, there is a general sense that we are not quite sure of what we are paying for, and except in some quite notable cases like AIDS, childhood leukemia, and organ transplantation—just to name the most prominent examples— the public (most often in the voices of insurers, government, and health maintenance organizations) is clamoring for a better justification of health-care costs. For instance, we are pleased to note the decline in heart disease and strokes (largely due to lifestyle changes), but why has the War on Cancer been in stalemate for 25 years, despite the billions of dollars spent on laboratory research?

As a scientist, I appreciate the magnitude of the problem and understand the nature of our slow progress, but as a health care consumer, I wonder if we have appropriately applied our resources. Perhaps more money should have been allocated to prevention and education, and less to the laboratory? We do not really know. And more fundamentally, we are not certain of the true efficacies of routine clinical practice. And as we shift from considering the best national policy for primary research goals to thinking about the immediacy of patient care, we feel similarly confused about whether we truly know how to make rational, cost-effective decisions.

The pragmatics of medical decision-making are complex indeed, and it is naive for a patient to think that any clinical decision is based simply on "the facts." Medical facts, like all other facts, reside in a complex context that requires interpretation and orientation. One can not simply apply a clinical datum to a particular scientific equation and find an "answer" popping out in the form of a therapy or diagnostic test. Medical logic comprises many different kinds of analysis and data. The evidence is gathered from different levels of research: (1) basic (i.e., laboratory-based), clinical, and epidemiologic studies, (2) randomized clinical trials, and (3) systematic reviews which attempt to offer the physician critically appraised synthesized results of primary investigations. More often than not, doctors must rely on this last kind of analysis to deal with the complex and myriad components that come into play in pointing to a "final" decision on how to deal with a particular clinical problem. These kinds of analyses, as well as textbook summaries, obviously reflect both good judgments as well as biases and misinterpretations. While such reviews and position papers written by panels of experts must inform clinical practice, by and large, their practical application is a matter for the individual, resting on one's personal experience and intellectual interpretation of these various sorts of distilled medical knowledge. Particular cases require individuating a patient within his or her proper cohort and weighing-in probablistic inference relevant to expected outcomes.

In other words, we play the odds—but we also follow our hunches. For example, I know an endocrinologist who frequently prescribes thyroid hormone to patients with "normal" thyroid function tests, because he believes that his clinical assessment is more valid than the existing laboratory data. And I not uncommonly have prescribed an anticancer drug to treat a disease for which that drug has not been formally approved—based on a guess that it will be effective. This is typical of modern practice.

Given the latitude in proper assignment, coupled with the general level of certainty in medicine which is reflected by heated controversies and admitted ignorance, it is no small wonder that the science of medicine is so often guided by intuition. Often referred to as "the art of medicine," the good physician's "artistic" gloss is taken to reveal the discrepancy between our aspirations for a rational, scientific (i.e., certain) medicine and an approximation of one.

A new field of medical assessment emerged in the 1980s to address the critical gap between our best medical knowledge and what comprises typical clinical care. It is generally understood that not all therapies or health care decisions that have been used are validated. The problem has many layers, spanning physician ignorance or conservatism, to resource or economic restrictions, to outright (but unavoidable) scientific ignorance. Specialists have recently appeared who have declared as their special mission the determination of assessing clinical evidence, that is, determining how strongly the data support a particular therapy or diagnostic procedure, and whether and how such intervention might be applicable to patients and under what conditions. This makes it sound as if such evaluations should have been standard practice in a science-based medicine—and it was. But in 1992, when this approach was dubbed "evidence-based medicine," we witnessed the birth of a new self-consciousness in the medical profession in answer to the increasing pressures for economic accountability. Replete with specialty journals devoted to this problem, special postgraduate courses to train physicians in its methods, and international collaborative studies to determine the efficacies of health care interventions, a new evaluative discipline emerged. The federal government, through the U.S. Agency for Health Care Policy and Research, has mandated support for this effort by approving research budgets devoted to projects concerned with obtaining efficacy data and other programs committed to disseminating evidence-based information on the clinical effectiveness in the management of important disorders. This movement is obviously stimulated by a concern with improving the efficiency of our health care budget, but there are deeper sources for these critical appraisals.

I believe this reassessment of the role of science in medicine reflects a growing sophistication of both the physician and the medical consumer, a realignment, resulting in higher expectations, of how we think about health and illness, and most fundamentally, about the nature of ourselves as humans. After all, our biological character, and more personally, our physical well-being, are largely informed by how and whether we perceive ourselves as sick or healthy. For at least four generations that identity was defined by a medicine based on science. But now there seems to be a growing awareness that science alone is an insufficient basis for clinical care. I am not referring to alternative medical therapies (certainly becoming more acceptable in social groups heretofore eschewing them), nor to exploiting Eastern-based philosophies of mind-body relationships (which until now were discerned solely by intuition and still have little scientific merit). I am rather alluding to a fundamental concern that laboratory-based medicine addresses only one component of being sick—namely, its materialistic aspect, which may be measured by physical or chemical means. Undoubtedly these scientifically based approaches are enormously powerful, but there are other dimensions of being ill that require attention. I am referring to the emotional and moral aspects of illness, that personal dimension to which science has little to contribute directly. We are happy to use science to develop new technologies, but at the same time we recognize that as the body is reduced to just so many materialistic parameters of measurement, the person inhabiting that body may be de-personalized, if not lost altogether. In the major overhaul that we call health care reform, the dollars and cents debates concerning costs and access to care have seemingly dominated the discussion. As complex as these economic issues might be, they are, in a sense, the simpler matter. The implicit question amid the many debates concerning medical economics is the issue of quality, and health care planners too often have been plagued by the seemingly impossible task of resolving concerns about cost, access, and quality into a coherent policy.

Undoubtedly, we can find various explanations of how and why American medicine is currently undergoing a major reorientation in economic, sociological, political, and cultural critiques. I have no doubt that these are crucial to our understanding, but I also believe that the dominant issue resides in how *we* regard ourselves when ill, and what *we* expect from the physician who cares for us. It is here that science still requires the "art" of the clinician. But the art of medicine is neither reimbursed, nor is it factored into health care costs. It is the hidden variable of caring and it is neglected at our peril. How science and its technology will figure in our future calculations of the health care budget—both in real dollars and in the more obscure calculus of quality—is informed by a general assessment of science's role in clinical care. To the historical development of that portion of the medical axis I now turn.

Antecedents

"Hello, Fred, this is John."

I had expected his call. Married to my cousin, he often asked me for medical advice or referrals. The day before he had narrated the long and painful story of my cousin's newly diagnosed pancreatic cancer. The malignancy had spread to the liver and her prognosis was grave. John had found an experimental protocol in Texas that promised astounding results. We had conferred and agreed that even a partial remission was worth every effort. It was appropriate to fly her to Houston.

"I called Texas and imagine, they refused to even look at Carol!"

"Why?"

"They wouldn't say. I think they simply didn't want a corpse lowering their results."

I couldn't respond. Flashing through my mind was the memory of my Uncle Barry going to the National Institutes of Health in the 1960s for an experimental protocol for his daughter, Judy, who had Hodgkins Disease. The chemotherapy, later proven to be the definitive regimen for her disease, was denied because Judy had already been treated with radiation therapy. A Dr. G. smugly told my uncle that she did not fulfill the protocol's criteria and she would not be enrolled. Uncle Barry started yelling and pounding the desk at which Dr. G. sat, facing the fury of my uncle. It must have been quite a scene, for Judy was indeed given the drugs.

Dr. G. went on to become one of the country's leading cancer researchers, celebrated in every quarter. Today Judy has three healthy children and lives happily in Vermont. Carol had no such luck. She died six weeks later.

Medicine as a clinical science was born in the hospitals of Paris during the French revolution. In a complex interplay between the reorganization of the medical establishment (resulting from the political upheaval) and the birth of biology as a new kind of examination of life processes, a new agenda was based on an attempt to establish rigorous scientific criteria for the natural history of disease and its etiology. Beginning with rigorous attempts to correlate anatomic pathology with clinical symptoms and signs, medicine became firmly affixed to the scientific agenda of establishing disease as an object of scientific dissection. By the 1820s, the physiologist Claude Bernard (1813–1878) adopted a stark objectivism to find the parameters of normal and pathological physiological function. Thus development of chemical analyses led to the field of physiology on the one hand, and correlation of clinical signs and symptoms to anatomic changes led to a new conception of pathology on the other. Their coupling transformed medicine from a descriptive discipline to a scientific one, generating the pathophysiological model still operative today.

By the 1840s, German physiologists led by Hermann Helmholtz (1821–1894) explicitly stated their scientific objectives: Physiology (and by extension, medicine) was to be reduced to physics and chemistry. This program was a deliberate attempt to purge vitalism from the science of life. In other words, biology would not seek any vestige of a postulated force unique to plants and animals that accounted for their peculiar vitality. Closely related to this materialistic program was the removal of any divinely authored design in creation, that is, teleology. Even before Charles Darwin (1809–1882) published *On the Origin of Species* in 1859, these scientists were explicitly committed to reducing the biological to the inorganic, seeking universal materialistic parameters of life processes. By measuring through careful quantitative techniques the amount of heat generated by contracting muscle, Helmholtz demonstrated the conversion and conservation of energy, and thus he strictly applied for the first time the laws of inorganic chemistry and physics to organic processes. The reductionists did not argue that certain organic phenomena were not unique, but only that all causes must have certain elements in common. They thus connected biology and physics by equating the ultimate bases of their explanations.

This new reductivist ethos was to govern the spectacular rise of medicine in the nineteenth and twentieth centuries; the influence of these European scientists cannot be overestimated. The principles they advocated were adopted in the U.S. through the Flexner Report of 1910, which served as the basis for accrediting medical schools that were committed to a scientific curriculum and licensing the physicians who graduated from them. Sponsored by the "orthodox" medical establishment based in the leading medical schools, this report served to fashion legislation that effectively ended the legitimacy of alternative medical theories and their practitioners. Aside from having a strong background in basic science, the new physician was to be taught that clinical medicine was but a branch of pathophysiology. The vector of interest was firmly drawn *from* the laboratory *to* the bedside. In other words, though clinical problems still framed medical research, the doctor was now trained as a basic scientist who would then apply his or her scientific skills to the clinical setting. The paragon became the sophisticated researcher; and the clinician immersed in anecdote and intuition, though still valuable where science had yet to advance, became a relic of a displaced medical folk art.

The challenge of laboratory-based medicine to bedside-oriented clinical practice was clearly discerned as a dangerous development in the opening decades of this century by such leading physicians as William Osler (1849–1919) and Francis Peabody (1881–1927). Osler was easily the most distinguished physician of his age. Author of a definitive textbook of medicine and a clinical leader of the newly established Johns Hopkins School of Medicine (an institution soon to become the premier model of academic medicine), he was a man who commanded respect from all quarters of the medical establishment. Peabody, likewise a distinguished physician, was Chief of Medicine of the Harvard service at the Boston City Hospital. Each saw the ascendance of this new scientific model as ruthlessly (and unnecessarily) sacrificing a humanistic element. They advocated a defense of the patient as sufferer and ward of the physician.

Osler essentially rejected the Flexner Report, warning against the appointment of medical faculty based on their research accomplishments as opposed to their interests in students and patients. Not only was he concerned with diverting students to the laboratory, but more so he worried that scientists would make poor physician role models and inadequate clinical teachers. He was not at all opposed to science applied to medicine, but he vigorously resisted a scientific ethos imposing itself between physician and patient. Peabody, similarly dismayed, warned that "the laboratory never can become and never should become the predominating factor in the practice of medicine." The question was of course basic to the physician's identity. Many, embracing the positivism of the age, rigorously contested the orientation advocated by Osler and Peabody, and the debate continued within the profession throughout the twentieth century.

Osler and Peabody eventually lost. The response of the U.S. medical community was to establish a new clinician-scientist hybrid, crossing the English model of hospital-based research with that of the German laboratory. In 1908, The American Society of Clinical Investigation advocated this ideal, and the newly created Rockefeller Institute served as a model for training the new physician-scientist. The flush of promise heralded by the advances in biomedicine during the period from roughly 1875 to 1910 inspired a scientific basis for medical training and practice. The Rockefeller Foundation promoted this approach to medical training, and after World War II, through the National Institutes of Health, the federal government subsidized an enormous commitment to this scientific program and its attendant approach to disease.

Despite the growth and unparalleled success in scientifically based medicine, there were deep concerns. These arose from the very roots of scientific medicine, because the respective agendas of medicine and physiology were not as consonant as they initially seemed. Science purports a detached relationship between the subject (scientist) and its object (patient). Although this positivist ideal is both psychologically and philosophically problematic, it nevertheless stands as a crucial pillar of scientific methodology. Within limits, detachment must remain a scientific standard to avoid contamination by subjectivity. After all, to observe nature dispassionately, with an objective eye and a mind detached from personal prejudice and prejudgment of any kind, is the essence of the scientific method. Most would agree that the rise of science has been measured by the success of this divorce of the subject and object. The product has been threefold: a mathematical abstraction of the material world, a description of nature more highly nuanced and complex than those depictions relying on personal interpretation, and a technology based on both. The interposed distance between observing scientist and the object of his scrutiny is the fundamental necessity of modern science. Medicine has obviously profited from that detachment, but at enormous human cost.

A profound irony emerged as medicine assumed its new legitimacy in laboratory-based science: the clinician lost his own boundaries and focus. No longer possessing its own theory, medicine sought its explanatory roots in other scientific disciplines. A medicine built up from its own principles, the care of the ill, was subsumed to a medicine based on science. Critics repeatedly have voiced concern that the progressive infusion of scientific knowledge and methods into medicine have not led inevitably to improved patient care. And some, like Alvan Feinstein in *Clinical Judgment* (1967), have argued that relying too heavily on the scientific medicine of the laboratory may actually distort the clinician's judgment, to the detriment of the patient. (This issue concerns the judgments required to ascertain the consistency and reliability of laboratory tests in the context of a particular patient's illness; because of false negative or false positive test results—not an inconsiderable proportion of clinical data—experience and clinical acumen are required to place the confounding, and often contradictory, information into proper perspective.) Feinstein's plea for a clinical science that would address medicine's specific requirements has yet to be seriously entertained. Instead, anatomy, physiology, microbiology, biochemistry, and genetics continue exclusively to define the basis of medical theory, to offer it their positivist criteria, and to regulate designations of disease—all this by sciences that in fact possess no norm.

The normative is a human category; in medicine, we establish categories of normal and pathological. To be sure, there are biological limits of physiological function, but there are also important boundaries of health and illness that are culturally determined. When Freud diagnosed "hysteria," he witnessed a set of signs and symptoms quite different from those we see today. In Japan, body odor is a sign of sickness; in Los Angeles, if you smell bad, you forgot your deodorant. In New York, if you have an upset stomach, you take an antacid, while your Parisian colleague who insists on a disturbance of his liver will take a glass of wine or, more often, a suppository. These are normative evaluations and responses; they reflect the pervasive importance of the fact that we project our own feelings onto our experience of disease.

The issue here is not that the particular cultural norm is "constructed" (and thus deserves deconstruction), but that the norm has a certain latitude and that health—or what is referred to as the norm—*cannot* be defined solely by physical and chemical measurements of bodily function. Chemistry and physics seek to establish an ordered explanation of the material universe. But to be normal is a subjective application of what we believe to be right, of how we should *feel*. If we can establish a physico-chemical explanation for that dysfunction, all the better for a materialistic therapy. But there is so much of everyday discomfort, disruption, and disquiet that cannot be so explained, or that falls beyond the hospital's test result. I am referring to several kinds of complaints that scientific medicine cannot at present address: borderline pathologies such as backache, where often times little pathology and no clear treatment is offered; chronic illnesses where conventional cure is usually lacking; nonpathologies and general "dis-ease" where reflexology and beauty therapy exemplify the sorts of therapies that attempt to relieve social or psychological discomfort.

As millions of Americans turn away from scientifically based medicine, they express their pragmatic concern with unmet expectations—no longer sacrosanct, the claims and promises of scientific medicine have become subject to ever-increasing scrutiny. In this reassessment of clinical science, the public articulates a growing general appreciation that contemporary medicine may not yet have achieved its full potential. They respond to medicine's failure to address many ailments by seeking "alternative" therapies. Because clinical science is still far more inexact than we too often would care to admit, and because there are, in any case, many limits to its application, why not visit the chiropractor, the acupuncturist, the homeopath, the herbalist? These are the pretenders to the throne of orthodox medicine, and they are doing quite well, thank you. Estimates indicate that we actually spend as much, or more, time and money on nonconventional medicine as we do on scientifically approved approaches. I am not advocating that scientific medicine simply embrace these unproven practices, but I am observing that Western medicine forfeits the confidence of an enormous subpopulation of the ill by condoning only a scientifically approved standard of care. Not surprisingly, we are beginning to witness a reappraisal of alternative medicines as new research seeks to scientifically assess their therapies, and some HMOs already pay for such. Whether out of cynicism or conviction, health care providers seem increasingly aware that a comprehensive medicine must embrace a plurality of approaches.

"Alternative medicine" seems to be growing in the face of undeniable advances of medical science. There is an air of paradox here that must have deep cultural sources. Some would argue that we are witnessing an antiscientific sentiment, a form of anti-intellectualism. I think that there may be insight in that assessment, but I am more interested in another explanation, namely, that there be some way, real or imagined, in which the personhood of the patient is better addressed in the alternative therapies. Although obvious, it must be stated anyway: Scientific medicine, and more pointedly scientific medical practitioners, do not and cannot use science to address the personal dimension of suffering. We can prescribe therapies to relieve pain, but that is the trivial rejoinder. I am referring instead to the mental anguish and anxiety of being sick. This sort of pain calls for empathy, and for a concern that only an ethic of caring can address. It calls for emotional support that recognizes both the individual's particular psychological needs, but which also factors in the broader contextual and cultural issues that must be understood to effectively treat illness. The ill person may be only partially understood by an analysis of his or her disordered structure or biochemistry. Peabody again serves as an eloquent voice of caution: Admitting the importance of the scientific approach to the patient, he nevertheless noted that "it is easy to overlook the fact that the application of the principle of science to the diagnosis and treatment of disease is only one limited aspect of medical practice." And then he threw down the gauntlet: "One of the essential qualities of the clinician is interest in humanity, for the secret of the care of the patient is in caring for the patient." His enjoinder is indeed the overarching mandate of medicine.

Such warnings, however, were quickly drowned out, and from the laws of physics and chemistry a new medicine soon arose. Powerfully, inexorably, we are its beneficiaries. By mid-twentieth-century, Osler and Peabody were regarded as voices from another era, and the voices of less influential patient advocates were muffled as the expected promises of biomedical science were enthusiastically embraced by the scientists and the public who supported them. But I believe we must return to the concerns voiced by Osler and Peabody—after all, their fears have indeed been realized. And, indeed, in the past twenty years a new ethos has clearly arisen.

When I claim that the confidence in science has ebbed since an earlier enthusiasm, I refer not only to a certain impatience concerning our progress against cancer and a host of other diseases, but rather to the realization that scientific understanding alone, where the patient becomes a diseased body, represents an inadequate approach to the ill person. Americans are ambivalent in their expectations of medicine. On the one hand, they demand that medical science be scientific, but at the same time they want a humane physician, not simply a technocrat, taking care of them. When the average American seeks medical attention, he or she expects that the full power and empirical effectiveness of scientific medicine will be applied for his or her benefit. On the other hand, that same patient recognizes an alarming reality in being subject to that power with resultant loss of control, fragmentation of the self, and the fracture of autonomy. Values central to our personhood are sacrificed as psychological payments for being cured. The extent to which the physician provides insulation and protection from that dehumanization has become an important component of the measure of his or her success. No one would wish to lessen medicine's enormous success as science, but fear of the power of science and of its alienation from humane values abides. Physicians must be more than brokers of science: they must also be ministering agents for the patient. These essentially complementary roles have long histories, penetrating our very characterization of the effective physician.

The Problem of a "New" Agenda

As we've already seen, a radical reassessment of medicine has occurred, where physicians no longer enjoy the autonomy once granted by their privileged status as priests of a scientific cult that enjoyed unbridled authority. Increasingly, their control of medicine has been wrested away, as they have been painstakingly scrutinized and criticized by paymasters and patients. This revolution in health care delivery is still incomplete, and we continue to wrestle with its most obvious manifestation, rationing the national health care budget and extending care to the uninsured. But already we witness a marked shift in the physician's role *vis à vis* the patient.

The conceptual foundations upon which this shift has occurred may be summarized: Medicine is now readjusting its views concerning subject-object relations. Today's physician can no longer view the suffering patient as an isolated object but must consider him or her within a far more complex panoply of suffering. The ideal health care provider now projects a set of personal concerns which must be incorporated into a complex set of judgments beyond the objective scientific data. These incorporate the idea of health as optimal function, longevity, vigor, and psychological adjustment, in short, all those parameters that fall into the newly comprehensive existential model of disease. In plain terms, the medical scientific model is simply too restricted to accommodate the cries of a public demanding ideal health. Thus the model of disease championed in the Flexner Report written at the beginning of this century hardly suffices to govern the medical profession today. Ironically, an older, more comprehensive role for the physician beckons, one based on the fundamental humane relationship between doctor and patient.

The gulf between medicine's technocratic advances and these newly rediscovered humane concerns manifests itself in many arenas, but perhaps most strikingly in the movement toward financial capitation. Here we witness the reassertion of the comprehensive responsibility of the physician for the health of the patient. No longer committed only to curing disease, crisis medicine has been replaced by the ancient Chinese practice, where the physician prospered only if his patient was well: payment would cease when illness occurred. Instead of being rewarded for performing procedures and prescribing therapies, the physician paid by capitation is rewarded in a sense for *not* treating the patient. Some critics consider that such a system would lead to shortcutting patient care, by allowing the dictates of a severely limited budget to justify withholding certain diagnostic procedures and therapies. Where previously the largess of the health care budget often permitted overzealous prescription, this system might easily err in the opposite direction. But optimists see this system's physician as committed to a comprehensive service which endeavors to keep the patient healthy and essentially out of trouble. Far from being ignored, the capitated patient (if the system works as advertised) would receive, as she does for her car or furnace, the full benefits of protective maintenance.

This debate is a classic case of rationing and risk taking, where too often the proponents and critics base arguments about policy on fragmentary data, unclear facts, and incompletely described outcomes. Whatever the final resolution, the final system will present new challenges and demands on the physician. Not only trained to treat disease, doctors will be required to know how to prevent illness, slow degeneration, promote safety, and counsel health in all its manifestations. To do so, the physician concerned with comprehensive health will need to be attentive to the patient not as an individual with a disease or disability, but as a person in the full exhibition of his or her personhood. This self-conscious attempt to treat patients comprehensively then becomes an important driving force for what has been billed as humanistic medicine, deeply self-aware of its ethics and its global responsibilities.

If such a reorientation indeed reflects fundamental shifts in our views of health and illness, then we should expect other signs of change. As I've already pointed out, not crisis management but health maintenance and prevention of illness have increasingly dominated current theoretical and general public discussions about how to distribute medical resources. Another arena in which an alternate ethos is taking hold concerns the scientific agenda that would guide medicine. We are witnesses to an important change of emphasis in clinical research: Although disease and the practice of defining it by fundamental scientific study retain a critical role in medical practice, the research agenda must now factor in new concerns.

The revolutionary changes in health care delivery must be understood as more than responses to the social, economic, and political pressures that have attempted to create a more cost-efficient delivery system. Beyond the obvious shifts in the industry's finances and organization, powerful revisions in medicine's dominant scientific agenda have initiated a cascade of changing attitudes and values among both consumers and health professionals. Because of the increasing centralization of economic power in government and large insurers, the boundaries of medicine have been reset. Medicine no longer enjoys its former relative autonomy as a self-governing scientific endeavor, having been forced to accommodate demands for health care delivery based on different principles. The repercussions of these changes are causing a crisis in medicine, because they have initiated a fundamental reorientation of the scientific agenda. Given the political power of this challenge, the older order has been shaken and forced to adapt quickly to new demands.

Funding by federal and private sources for basic research continues to grow, but the public is increasingly concerned with the practical application of medical expertise, both in its delivery to all segments of society and its cost-effectiveness. An excellent example of how research might be politicized is the increasing attention given to women's health issues. In 1991 the National Institutes of Health launched a $600 million study called the Women's Health Initiative. It was designed to examine the effects of a low fat diet, hormone therapy, and vitamin and calcium supplements on heart disease, cancer, and osteoporosis in women. The project is so large and comprehensive that it has been described as "almost like a military campaign." And well it might, for it represents a national consensus that greater attention must be paid to women's health concerns, and no less than a massive assault is required to get the data. Another related case is the growing attention paid to breast cancer. Critics correctly noted that relative to the public health problem, research devoted to breast cancer was modest, to say the least. In the past decade outreach programs for screening mammograms, funding for large-scale clinical trials, and increased basic research support are each elements of a deliberate response to strong public criticism that women's health issues have received too little attention. Whereas an investigator might argue for exploring the genetic, biochemical, or biophysical basis for malignancy, we now see that support has become, in many instances, both large scale (at the expense of smaller grants to individual scientists) and goal directed, identifying a specific agenda. For better or for worse, at the very least we are witnessing science—no longer seemingly insulated from its social foundations—being forced to become more responsive to its supporting political context. Activists demand that their own priorities be addressed, and in response, the veils of an esoteric research program are pushed aside by citizen scrutiny. Naderism has extended to the health care industry. In short, a better educated public has asserted that science is too important to be left to the scientists alone, and the laboratory is now subject to external influence, if not control.

The political pressures on medicine have been driven by both the growing "contextualization" of science (the public's demand for accountability) and the economic restrictions on the health care industry that would specify the distribution of limited resources. Throughout the process of reallocating capital, a more holistic, patient-oriented approach has arisen to counterbalance the opposing drives for a more fundamental, reductionist scientific approach to disease. This is not to say that the former orientation is either antiscientific or unscientific, only that its program is based on a wider agenda: In addition to careful analyses of cost-effectiveness, the more humanistic concerns represent a response to the call to assign resources for more comprehensive health delivery—both scientific and compassionate. Thus I hasten to add that it is not incommensurable for a reductionist, laboratory-based investigator to be as well a compassionate physician in the clinic. But by and large, we do indeed have two competing programs that seek to dominate medical practice. These two agendas, one of the pragmatics governed by the market place and the other of the deeper humane commitments of the discipline, have clashed, rigorously competing to establish the boundaries and conceptual goals of medicine. We are now beginning to witness the practical results of that conflict.

"Why haven't you given me a draft of that paper? Jackson published his abstract . . . we'll be scooped. We have to submit to the journal by next week."

"I"m sorry, but I got caught up in clinic yesterday, and then I had night call."

"Poor excuse. Never allow patient care to interfere with your career."

My priorities were clear. The admonishment stung. I knew the lesson well. At the end of my internship my chief resident pulled me aside and confided, "Fred, you'll be a full professor before any of us, but please, don't bother caring for patients!" I was miffed, but he was perceptive and I knew his insight was correct. Only years later was I to reassess my priorities.

My early training required a major overhaul.

I am a scientist. I trained as a biochemist and I spent the better part of my formative years as a physician in the laboratory. Success as a basic researcher assured my rapid climb up the professorial ladder. I learned the key lessons for academic advancement from a mentor at Harvard, himself a highly productive researcher, who in my opinion contributed more to the welfare of the public than one hundred—or for that matter, one thousand—ordinary clinicians, if any such comparison could be made. But that career model, whether translated into the prosaic concerns of doctors making money or academics wishing to rise in the medical school hierarchy, must strike most patients as callous, even severely selfish. Different models of excellence clearly have their place, but in the setting of the clinic, the patient is concerned with his or her own care, not the self-aggrandizement of the doctor. Yet the rewards in our medical schools do not traditionally go to the teacher or the committed clinician, but rather to the competitive clinician-scientist, dedicated to (depending on your point of view) the expansion of knowledge, or more cynically, the accrual of grants, prestige, and overhead dollars for the university. In either case, under the rubric of science, the medical establishment has almost universally (until quite recently) rewarded the successful researcher at the expense of the clinician. But now the standards are beginning to change. Why?

Perhaps the clearest sign of science's retreat as the governing, if not exclusive, ethos for medicine and its replacement by this more self-conscious concern for the patient as person is the growing movement of patient rights. Modern medical ethics was born of a basic suspicion that physicians were perhaps neither so omniscient nor infallible in their fiduciary actions as the public might hope. Most commentators would mark the birth of contemporary medical ethics with the legal assertion of patients' rights as enunciated in the famous Quinlan case of 1975. Robert Morse, a young attending physician, and Joseph Quinlan, the father of the comatose twenty-one year old woman, Karen, contested the right to terminate her care. The Quinlans based their decision to cease support on Pope Pius XII's 1958 pronouncement concerning cases such as theirs. On this Catholic opinion, the rights and duties of the family depended on the presumed will of the patient, resuscitation was not a necessary obligation, and if resuscitation (writ large) was a burden to the family, they might lawfully insist on discontinuation of care. Their doctor opposed the request of the family based on his interpretation of medical precedent and state law, and in the resulting civil case, the New Jersey Supreme Court upheld the parents' position by ruling Karen's affirmed "independent right of choice" or "self-determination", as a constitutional "right to privacy." The family could exercise this right on her behalf if there was no reasonable possibility of her emerging from the coma. The Court added the condition that an "Ethics Committee" concur with the decision, and thus was born the universal requirement for such an institution.

Although the Quinlan case clearly established the rights of patients to refuse life-sustaining treatment, the deeper moral implication validated critiques of what was then conventional medical ethics: While physicians were authoritative about medical *facts*, they were not necessarily expert or autonomous regarding *moral principles* or *values*. The central ethical issue was not to uphold what might be understood as medically indicated or acceptable, but rather to adjudicate "Whose values decide?" The Quinlan case fundamentally held that decisions concerning medical care were situated firmly within the patient's autonomous domain, and scientific expertise could not be extended beyond its proper quarter. With various forms of medical "paternalism" thus discounted, the 1970s and 1980s witnessed the championing of self-determination with all of its attendant supports.

As David Rothman has documented in *Strangers at the Bedside*, physicians are now accompanied by vigilant medical ethicists, eager lawyers, nervous hospital administrators, and suspicious patients, each of whom is concerned to maintain the fine boundaries protecting patient autonomy. But traditionally this claim to individual rights has been counterpoised to the interests of the community as a whole, so that the issue of respecting the needs of the individual must be balanced with the often conflicting common interests of the body politic. This theme has had diverse enactments since Antigone buried her brother against the orders of the king, and we, quite naturally, continue to debate the balance between libertarian aspirations of American individualism and our countervailing communitarian morality.

When this issue is discussed in the context of medical ethics, we find the same general outlines of the debate. Some have argued that the comprehensive foundation for the ethical framework of medicine should be posited not on the principle of autonomy, but rather on the "principle of permission." This principle privileges not some abstract value like autonomy or liberty, but rather a secular moral authority guided by the common consent of the whole group. Morality thus becomes relational, a contract between consenting individuals seeking a common good. In this construction, *relation* is critical, and the autonomy of the respective individuals subordinate. This is not to sacrifice autonomy, but rather to shrink it appropriately, to treat it as one factor among many in the relations between citizens.

This understanding of definition by relation has played an important role in twentieth-century philosophy, as scathing critiques have eroded the idea of autonomy, the governing principle of moral philosophy since the Enlightenment. This reassessment originated in an even more fundamental conceptual revolution, within which the autonomous self has come to be seen as only a step in the evolution of our ideas about what is human. I refer here to the comprehensive question of *selfhood*. The cardinal issue is to situate humankind in its existential context, not as autonomous individuals living freely and alone, but embedded in the world. The general theme I wish to expound is that a person is not a self-contained entity, self-defined or in any sense independently "established," but he rather becomes authenticated in his encounters with others, whether physical, social, or divine. Later theorists, often referred to as postmodernists, regarded the self as arbitrarily structured on an edifice composed by particular cultural and historical encounters. So not only was the self seen as devoid of boundaries or a constituted essence, but its very construction was a contingency—and a radical one at that. Let me briefly review the history of this philosophical view, for in elucidating our radically shifting sense of selfhood, we encounter the underlying problematics of medical ethics.

2

The Course of Autonomy

Autonomy in Medicine

Joe was a close friend. Fifteen years older than I, he was like an older brother, someone who gave good counsel and comforted me in many settings. At age 59 he had quit his university job and was enjoying the fruits of a modest and satisfying retirement. His wife adored him, and he had many friends. Joe had a comfortable life.

One morning he called. "Doc, I don't feel so well."

"What's wrong?"

"I'm not sure. Sort of feel nauseated; can't eat."

Joe was no complainer. "I'll be right over."

When I arrived, Joe was lying on the couch. He looked pale. I took his pulse. It was irregular and faint. "I don't like this. Sarah, call an ambulance."

When we arrived at the emergency room, the intern took an electrocardiogram and returned with the tracing. "Looks like an acute MI."

"What?" Joe asked incredulously.

"A heart attack." Turning to me the young doctor said, "Look, we have to act quickly. The infarct seems restricted to the inferior pole. We have a protocol for various clot busters. What do you want to do?"

I turned to Joe. "Listen, we can either treat you with standard methods or try some new therapies that open up clogged blood vessels. They are designed to aid in dissolving the clot blocking your coronary artery."

"What do you think?" Joe asked expectantly.

"I'm not sure what's best. If we knew, there would be no experimental protocol. I'll discuss this with the cardiologist."

I paged Dr. C., and while waiting for him, quickly reviewed the proto-
col, some 25 pages of experimental background, preliminary clinical data,
expected complications, and the like. I was no expert in heart disease, so
I was much relieved to speak with Dr. C., who explained in three sentences
the expected complications and what he thought were relatively low risks.
I returned to Joe.

"I don't know what to say, really. The doctors here are enthused about
this new protocol, but who knows. At least with the standard regimen we
know the likely outcomes." These I briefly explained, and Joe looked at
Sarah and asked, "Well honey, what do you think?"

She shrugged her shoulders. He looked at me and said, "Doc, you
decide."

"Enroll in the protocol." The intern overhearing this conversation ran
out of the room and quickly returned with the permission paperwork. Joe,
hooked up by now to I.V.s and monitors, stripped of his clothes, with
nurses and doctors running around his stretcher, scribbled his signature
and closed his eyes. They whisked him up to the intensive coronary care
unit and began infusing the medication—which one, no one knew because
the vials were coded. The study was double-blinded so that neither the
patient nor the doctors and nurses were aware which drug was being deliv-
ered.

Six hours later, Joe suffered a massive bleed into his brain. Surgery failed
and he died the next morning.

Thus far I have discussed the state of medicine as one in flux, with a historical trajectory of scientific medicine having led to disquiet regarding how
we care for the ill. I am of course also interested in the various social and
economic factors at play today, but my primary task is of a different kind.
While my thesis must be placed within a cultural context at a particular
historical moment, the questions raised by the current crisis in medicine
demand in addition another kind of inquiry: a philosophical discussion,
which by its very nature addresses the broadest issues relevant to our predicament. In this chapter I begin to erect a philosophical argument that
attends to the question at hand, namely, How might we establish medicine
to better fulfill its humane concerns? To locate the philosophical undercur-
rents at play might enable us to identify the social and technological winds

buffeting us. With a clearer notion of our ethical expectations of medicine, perhaps we can articulate a program of medical reform, from education to economic prioritization, from technological applications to guidelines for care. In short, with a keener appreciation of the deepest philosophical issues that so powerfully inform our worldviews and our understanding of ourselves, we will have an effective tool by which to assess our medical industry and redirect it so that it serves us more adequately.

Philosophers talk of "grounding" ethics. This is their vernacular for trying to establish the foundations of a moral philosophy. Given the endless debates, this is surely an ongoing and incomplete task. In large measure the grounding problem arose when secularism began to eclipse theology. When religion determined conduct, revelation and interpretation of the Divine Word definitively dictated morality. At the dawn of the modern age, theology was overtaken by different kinds of knowledge, and revelation no longer would offer us an ethical pole star by which we might orient our lives. Science helped formulate this new way of thinking, and in turn secularism supported the growth of science. In this mutual relationship, science became a major beneficiary of secularism, and secularism used science to support its war against the religious domination of civil life. Medicine, accordingly, was transfigured by the growth of science, and its ethical structure was concomitantly changed.

It is no easy matter to adjudicate even a common basis by which we might discuss ethics in medicine. Aside from some powerful religious traditions which still command respect and response, arguments of contemporary American secularism tend to alternate between a pragmatic utilitarianism and a more kindred religious orientation now based on natural law. In each case, our ethics emulate a democratic ideal and attend to the pluralistic demands of a diverse society composed of multiple ethnic and religious allegiances. But in different political contexts other ethical ideals can and do arise. For instance, we might base our ethics on a Greek ideal, on notions of the Good or the Excellent. Or we might seek a universal relational morality in which a sense of responsibility for another resides in some other kind of understanding, for instance in our biological natures as communal animals, or perhaps in a universal religious construction. Thus ethics in this age of an acute awareness of diverse cultural practices has become, in some sense, another forum for seeking consensus between

competing philosophical orientations. So in our discussion, the more pertinent question becomes: How might we ground medical ethics in philosophy at large?

Contemporary medical ethics was largely born in the attempt to rescue
the patient's dignity from the gross manipulation and dehumanization of
a technologically driven clinical science. The discontent that seemed to
underlie all the various criticisms stemmed from a concern for patient
autonomy, the moral notion most easily extrapolated from the legal precepts of our political culture. From those critiques the anthem reached a
crescendo in the 1970s, in the demand that patients should lose none of
their rights as autonomous individuals simply because of their illness. They
were entitled to read their medical charts, know their diagnoses, participate
in therapeutic decisions, and decide how they would die, if it came to that.
Perhaps the most radical expression of this sentiment was the extension
of such rights to institutionalized patients suffering from mental illness.
Thomas Szasz and other psychiatric activists of the 1960s led the movement to emancipate these patients from mental hospitals. Not even the
deranged were to be freed from their autonomy. Unless considered dangerous to themselves or others, they were unfettered to roam the streets and
fend for themselves as best as they could. Now, we can see them daily,
muttering to themselves, pushing shopping carts and lugging grocery bags
full of their belongings.

I would hardly argue against patient autonomy. But I do doubt that it
is a sufficient foundation upon which we might build a more humanistic
medicine. I have come to that conclusion based on a philosophical analysis that seeks to establish the fundamental descriptive terms of medical
ethics. When I invoke philosophy, I am not attempting to argue some
formalistic doctrine, full of technical jargon and subtle distinctions. Philosophy is the proper forum for this discussion because it claims the overarching ability to articulate the many relevant issues: We need a
description of medical practice that responds to current demands but
which may, at the same time, guide us in the moral dimension of medicine. The business of philosophy is to analyze. It rarely if ever "solves"
its problems in the way that, say, an engineer solves the design of a bridge
over a particular chasm, or a businessman solves the delivery problem to
an outpost in Mongolia.

These issues have a long history, and I will first briefly trace some of those antecedents, not so much to offer a history lesson, but to help frame how we think of ourselves as "selves." We begin here because the notions of personhood and morality are intimately entwined throughout our understanding of moral agency. Our conceptions of the individual have changed dramatically since the seventeenth century, and ethics is now based on a particular conception of how persons should act; we must now seek an integrated philosophy—of self and ethics—appropriate to our own time and place. I would not dispute the successes of ethics based on autonomy born three centuries ago, but I am intent on demonstrating the limitations of that political idea for contemporary medicine. Autonomy has certainly served a critical function in the evolution of liberal society, but it was an invention, a construct of a particular time and place, and as we know, time takes no holiday. So let us now review how the idea of autonomy grew in its own historical context, and its fate in philosophy.

The Birth of Liberal Autonomy

Out of the night that covers me
Black as the Pit from pole to pole,
I thank whatever gods may be
for my unconquerable soul.

In the fell clutch of circumstance,
I have not winced, nor cried aloud:
Under the bludgeonings of chance
My head is bloody, but unbowed.
. . .

It matters not how strait the gate,
How charged with punishment the scroll,
I am the master of my fate;
I am the captain of my soul.

—William H. Henley, *Invictus*

The liberal notion of individual rights originated with British democracy, which itself arose from a complex interplay of economic, social, political, and intellectual currents of the seventeenth century. Among the philosophical builders who erected supports for this political agenda, John Locke (1632–1704) is credited as being a key architect, constructing a philosophy that provided the conceptual edifice for the political and legal expression of those ideals. Locke was well situated to learn the practicalities of science and medicine, as well as their philosophical basis, by apprenticing with the foremost leaders of each discipline. From Robert Boyle (1627–1691) he studied physical experimental methods and the theory upon which they were based, and from Thomas Sydenham (1624–1689), the greatest physician of the early modern period, he learned medicine. But rather than becoming a natural philosopher, one committed to studying nature, Locke devoted himself to politics and diplomacy, and it was in that arena that he applied the lessons he learned from the scientists and physicians of his circle.

A self-consciousness among scientists of the period grew from a concern about how our perceptions determine our knowledge of the world and how our minds influence our perceptions. These early scientists well appreciated that rationality (our cognitive functions) and empiricism (our perceptual faculties) are interwoven in such complex ways that separating the two is impossible. As much as one might want to perceive the world objectively with no projection of prejudice or subjectivity, it is literally impossible to do so. At the same time, it became clear that description and experimentation demand just such a divorce, because the scientific method was ostensibly based on a scrupulous objectivity in which the observer would simply report his data and draw the logical inferences. Thus observer-autonomy was a key precept of the nascent scientific method, and philosophers struggled to establish the basis on which claims of objective knowledge could be made.

The problem of autonomy migrated from the laboratory to the political arena and became central to Locke's philosophy. Throughout the Enlightenment philosophers continued to wrestle with both the implications and the philosophical basis of his position, which pervaded both the judicial and the scientific discussion of this period. For Locke the political theorist, autonomy served as a crucial, one could say *the* critical fulcrum for a society struggling to transform itself from the subject of the divine rule of monarchs to self-government ruled by the democratic rights of the individual, seen as both the sole agent of his pursuit of happiness and arbiter of the social will. Violent revolutions in England, France, and America had effected this transition by the end of the eighteenth century.

Today we take for granted our autonomy; we think of ourselves as persons entitled to assert our individuality and choice. The history of this idea is fascinating, but the important point—and this is the critical philosophical caveat—is that the autonomous individual was *invented*. One may argue about natural being, God-given rights, or whatever other conceptual support there may be for the construct, but essentially, *homo democratus* emerged within English liberalism. Let me take a moment to summarize how this invention was formulated by Locke, the key author of this new political citizen. There are many interesting historical parallels and cross-currents in this issue relevant to constructing the appropriate moral domain for contemporary medicine.

Locke was deeply affected by the scientific achievements of Sir Issac Newton. Newton too emphasized *autonomy* as pivotal to his epochal discoveries of the laws of motion and gravity. The extraordinary power of his predictions had ordered the entire physical world, from falling apples to the firing of cannon balls, through simple equations of gravitational and mechanical forces. With this triumph of science, a particular kind of radically objectified, mathematically based characterization of the universe presented humankind with a revolutionary reassessment of its place in the world. In devising a mechanical and materialistic explanation of the motions of the heavenly bodies, human beings came to recognize themselves as possessing a new power to discern the mysteries of nature, and perhaps even themselves, through thought. The reasons for this basic reconsideration of our own human cognitive capacities are obviously terribly complex but may be summarized at least in one respect: With the scientific revolution, we became capable of observing nature and discerning its workings not by reason alone as the medieval scholastics had attempted, nor by some magical formula as the alchemists had endeavored, nor by divine revelation as the medieval church asserted, but by a novel approach, the empirical, objective "scientific method."

The scientific method resulted from a deliberate rationality of two kinds: proving a hypothesis—deduction—and generalizing from observations—induction. Data were collected and then organized according to their common features; this inductive process was coupled with the deductive logic of proposing a hypothesis and then either disproving it (thereby requiring a new hypothesis) or finding new support for its dominance. Science then was an innovative synthesis of logic and empiricism, a combination of "top-down" (hypothetico-deductive) and "bottom-up" (inductive) procedures. In each, empirical evidence and experimentation were used to garner abstract, mathematical characterizations of the physical world. For this method to work, the scientist had to attain a perspective on the world from an autonomous point of view, where prejudice played no role. The success of science depended on autonomy—of perception and of thought. This idea of man as aperspectival grew out of the invention of this scientific method, and both profoundly influenced much more than the laboratories and observatories of Europe.

The scientific ideal—unfettered rationality, objective experimentation, autonomous observation—translated into the political and moral ideals of seventeenth-century England. Locke's philosophy hinged upon the ability of the individual to detach himself from the world, indeed from his very self, and observe each objectively, just as Newton regarded apples falling and planets orbiting. The individual then becomes an independent consciousness, albeit a consciousness relating to the world through "objectivity." Self-conscious efforts to be objective dominated the birth of modern science, and it was this same concern for establishing the independence of a thinking subject—now with attendant legal rights—that dominated Locke's own thinking of the political, moral agent.

This emergence of the Lockean individual had profound ethical ramifications. The mode of objective disengagement in science became a moral requirement in scrutinizing not only the world but also the self. On the moral plane, these concepts were wedded to Locke's political philosophy, in which autonomy becomes a value, limited only to the extent that one individual's freedom infringes upon the freedom of others. The individual so defined becomes a basic unit of government, divided between his freedom and the rights of the majority. "Self" transmutes to a forensic term to which the law is applicable, and individuality is thus celebrated, and moreover, assured as established by this system of thinking which gives rise to an independent ethical unit. We are heir to seventeenth-century liberalism, and its view of Man as the essential proprietor of his or her own person.

Beyond this legal definition of the individual, the self became the focus of philosophical speculation as the "knowing" entity. The growing consciousness of the individual as observant creature seeking objective knowledge of the world led to basic questions about the very nature of the mind. How do we in fact separate ourselves as observers from the world, and by what means might we construe the mind that knows the world and itself? The best articulation of this epistemological agent, the one endowed with the capacity to know, was offered by Immanuel Kant (1724–1804) at the end of the eighteenth century, in what he called, "the transcendental apperception of the ego." By "transcendental" he meant that such an entity must exist as an *a priori* and necessary condition of experience as determined by the constitution of the mind itself. It just seemed both obvious and necessary that we have such a self for psychological cohesiveness.

Whereas Locke had extended the problem of selfhood to the political domain, Kant was more concerned with the problem of establishing a philosophical basis for the knowing entity. Although there were important moral implications of Kant's transcendental ego, the unification of our thought and experience commanded his attention. This construction was to a large extent an operational definition of selfhood, namely the sense of an inner, fundamental, and unchanging unity of our consciousness. For Kant some structured unity of consciousness—pure ego—precedes (and transcends) the content of our perceptions and makes possible their experienced order and meaning. Thus an entity—the self—was thought to be the necessary condition for having experience and for synthesizing that experience into a unity. In this manner, "personhood" assumed a particular definition of what was required to be a knowing entity.

This belief in a transcendent self served as the modernist basis for sense perception (how we know the world), for our definition of a political-legal unit of government (the citizen), for our emotional sense of identity (the psyche), and perhaps most fundamentally, for our conception of our very agency—our concept of who we *are*. From the mid–seventeenth century through the Kantian project, the self offered a perspective on the world and ordered it, thus becoming the locus of certainty and truth. For Descartes, Locke, Kant, and thinkers of their period, the self was an *entity*, something that cohered and was defined in such a way that met their philosophical and psychological needs. Charles Taylor, in *Sources of the Self*, wrote of this view of selfhood as "punctual," reflecting the idea that there was, in the vast plenum of experience, a kernel of identity that could not be further reduced or eliminated.

The most influential philosophy of the self in the twentieth century that followed this orientation was that of Sigmund Freud, who was very much committed to the concept of the self as an integrative whole, constituted by various layers of consciousness. The particularities of his theory are not critical for our discussion, but I might simply note that his analyses of dreams and everyday language and behavior postulated a self composed of several psychic categories, which nevertheless assumed a coherence of personality, hierarchically unified. We must not confuse his radical restructuring of the everyday ego by an underlying instinctual matrix in the unconscious as *philosophically* revolutionary. This is not to minimize the importance of his suggestion that we are ultimately governed by passions and aggressions scarcely contained by our moral superegos, but rather to recognize that in Freud's dethroning of the rational ego, the self as entity remained, only now more complex and mysterious. Despite this formulation—only apparently iconoclastic—Freud was very much an Enlightenment thinker, committed to a traditional notion of selfhood. His theory largely remained anchored in a modernist conception, namely that a self, perhaps dynamic in composition and action, nevertheless constituted an identity—an entity—with structure and boundaries.

Whether or not we are Freudians, most of us think that we are indeed "selves," that we have some protected, knowable inner identity to which we must cling in all of our dealings with the world—and for that matter, with our own psyches. Psychoanalysis was committed to defining such a self, to stabilizing it, and to rationalizing its anomalies. Its critical project, like that of Kant, was to find coherence, a narrative that would bestow some consistency or wholeness to the rational quest for personal identity. Those without a firm sense of self are fairly viewed as deranged, and we certainly cannot function in a social universe without some firm commitment to personal identification.

But this view of the self as a cohesive entity is too simple, and in its simplicity, it is false.

Perhaps an analogy will illustrate the problem. Let us say that we are driving to Boston. The sign says that we are sixty miles from the city, roughly an hour away. For various reasons, mainly the need to standardize distances, define boundaries, and the like, there is indeed a marker in Boston designating the heart of the city. For purposes of the sign on the highway, this marker *is* Boston. But I know Boston when I am in the city, and it is long before I reach the city marker that I feel the municipality in its diverse and multifold manifestations. In fact, I rarely even visit the vicinity of that city marker at all. It is in this sense a fictional spot, and for our discussion it is almost fully analogous to Locke's punctual self. But a key difference distinguishes them: Boston indeed has a central dot defined by its city government; I, as a self, have no such punctuated point of identity. What would such a point *be*? How might one even describe such a simile?

Nevertheless, we think of ourselves as selves. It is a most useful construct for the way we think of our personhood and our communal culture. But the historical record is plain: Each era has posited its own version of the person. The punctual self is the product of the Enlightenment and was constructed to deal with the particular philosophical challenges bequeathed by the political and social demands of that culture. We live in a different era, governed by a host of new cultural forces, and thus unsurprisingly our own notions of selfhood—defined by a long and complex, if not tortuous, historical development—are radically other than, for instance, Locke's or Kant's. Vestiges of their ideas surely remain, but other notions of selfhood have replaced these Enlightenment ones. We are embedded in our own time, and our period has substituted a version of the knowing subject distinct from that prescribed by the great thinkers living two, three, or four centuries ago. We might derive valuable insights from them, but the project of defining ourselves never ceases and the fundamental category of personhood is highly sensitive to changing context. In the following section I will summarize a radically different notion of the autonomous self, and then in the next chapter show how this entire conception has been challenged and overturned, with far-reaching moral consequences.

The Organic Self

The awakened and knowing say: body am I entirely, and nothing else; and soul is only a word for something about the body. The body is a great reason, a plurality with one sense, a war and a peace, a herd and a shepherd. . . . Behind your thoughts and feelings, my brother, there stands a mighty ruler, an unknown sage—whose name is self. In your body he dwells; he is your body.
—Friedrich Nietzsche, *Thus Spake Zarathustra*, "In the Despisers of the Body"

I introduced myself to philosophy when I was fourteen. In that age of awakening, I sought answers to the typically difficult—and, as I later understood, unanswerable—questions that have troubled metaphysicians over the ages. I began with two surveys: Will Durant's *The Story of Philosophy* and Bertrand Russell's *A History of Western Philosophy*. Despite the few, largely unsympathetic pages devoted to Friedrich Nietzsche (1844–1900), I was drawn to him. Why? I suppose in large part because he so clearly articulated the problems of selfhood that preoccupied my own quest for identity. Although usurped and thus compromised by Nazi ideology after his death, he provided something crucial for my own understanding of culture, ethics, rationality, and the self. He was like a lone timber wolf, wandering the dark forests of Europe and baying at the moon. He certainly did not fulfill the image I had of a rationalistic, analytic philosopher. In many ways he was a poet, celebrating our organic character. For me, he thus resided more comfortably in the pantheon of Walt Whitman, Dylan Thomas, and D. H. Lawrence, than in that edifice housing Socrates, Descartes, and Kant. Nietzsche unabashedly sought his roots and found them not in a social morality, but in a self-affirming assertion of his biological will. He was a perpetual teenager, and I recognized a kindred spirit when I encountered him! In fact, I was so contaminated by his temper that I chose not to take a single philosophy course in college. Although I read from Plato to Wittgenstein, I always returned to Nietzsche.

My devotion to Nietzsche was indeed well placed, perhaps not so much as a foundation for classical philosophy, but as a basis for understanding contemporary culture more broadly. Many roads into twentieth-century thought may be traced back to him, including our ideas of the unconscious, the pluralism of experience, the self-responsibility of morality, the role of art. In each domain, Nietzsche sought "self-authenticity," which ultimately depended on recognizing our biological nature and its full attainment in what he called "rapture." His was a romantic inquiry, and I believe that much of his message of how we might re-enchant our world with meaning, albeit individually derived and experienced, is a crucial statement of our collective aspirations. I have become highly critical of his formulation, but I recognize that to understand Nietzsche is to open an important window through which we view ourselves.

In my discussion of Nietzsche, I want to explicate two issues: The first concerns his notion of autonomy, one that was developed in our own post-Darwinian era; the second concerns "ideality," specifically the aspiration for ideal health and well-being that so marks our contemporary preoccupation with medicine. I believe that the way we think of ourselves, namely, as bodies, in fact as biological organisms, is a relatively new idea and that Nietzsche's conception of struggle and ideal health articulated sharply what has become a commonly held belief about the self. As useful as these notions are for many of our current views of health, another aspect of Nietzsche's thought is less helpful. This is the cul-de-sac into which the principle of autonomy situates ethics. Thus we will climb the Nietzschean mountain, take in the views, and descend so that we might ascend to another vantage point.

Nietzsche and nihilism seem to go hand in hand. This is a confusing issue, but simply put, Nietzschean nihilism comes in two modes. On the one hand, he attacked Western culture—and more specifically, Judeao-Christian morality. Leaving nothing sacrosanct and proclaiming "God is dead!" he launched an assault that was total and comprehensive. This "negative" nihilism prevails in Nietzsche's popular caricature, as something like the philosophical analogue to Sherman's March to the Sea. But there is a second kind of nihilism in Nietzsche's thought, one perhaps more subtle and elusive because of its lack of formal structure. This is the "positive" nihilism that espouses individual, at the expense of collective, morality. In deconstructing life's categories—whether social, psychic, historical, or moral—Nietzsche nevertheless expounds a radically personal ethics. Thus he replaced masks of illusion—ruthlessly exposing the treachery of belief in a foolproof, universal, and unshakable morality "out there"—with comprehensive self-responsibility, a nihilistic assertion that the self resides *in*, and *of*, and *by* itself.

In celebrating individual self-aggrandizement of our autonomous selves—a formulation indebted to Darwinism—Nietzsche founded his philosophy on the notion that personal responsibility for overcoming weakness, physical as well as moral, was the prime expression of our biological nature. That we might be perfected by exertion of our will was a philosophy that celebrated the individual and his (given Nietzsche's misogynist tendencies, he really meant *his*) full attainment. This links the overarching moral issue to the biological characterization and serves to integrate his thought.

Although in normal parlance the self usually has a certain permanency, an implicit stable configuration, certain nineteenth-century critiques destabilized this idea. Here I wish to emphasize, of the many sources that gave birth to the idea of the self's indeterminacy, the advent of evolutionary thinking in biology. This greatly influenced Nietzsche's thinking in particular, and it reoriented the general intellectual consensus on the nature of all organisms, human beings included. The blind materialism of Darwinian evolution pushed divine order onto the ropes of contingency and chance, thus undermining the theological presumption of a predestined order of the universe. Gone was the rationale for our very existence as a species. Absent teleology, what purpose can our being, *human* being, have? If all is accidental, then we are fundamentally a product of blind chance. In this setting, the punctual self, the product of a world view wherein stable entities made up the cosmos, wobbled. Change is of the essence—entities are in flux, essentially impermanent, and thus elusive.

Nietzsche was particularly sensitive to the implications of this Darwinian insight, and he correctly perceived the metaphysical implications of a radical, materialistic theory of evolution. Today the notions of change, progress, and ideality are indelibly imprinted on Western consciousness, but in the nineteenth century this metaphysical construction was tempered by a different sense of order. Darwinism dismissed once and for all the Aristotelian notion of essence, the idea that everything has some unchanging core identity. If *everything* is evolving, what remains essential or permanent? Nothing—and we have been forced to abandon the task of seeking essences as regulative identities. Not that we are necessarily comfortable with this new understanding—the older metaphysics remains deeply embedded in our culture, language, and philosophy—but the challenge remains, and we see many manifestations of its effects.

This metaphysics of change has had its deconstructive effect on our implicit understanding of our personhood; although the notion of the "Self" remains tenaciously embedded, we are self-consciously aware that to ask, What is the *essence* of our selfhood? is to ponder an inanswerable question. We cannot point to some character or behavior and say, *that* is the Self. We are left inarticulate and baffled by the query. Identity is only conferred by the continued evolution from some earlier manifestation. I look at photographs from different junctures of my life—as a baby, in high school, at medical school graduation, with my children—and I see widely divergent personae. But indeed those photographs do capture a person variously referred to as "Freddy," "Fred," "Dr. Tauber," "Dad." What . makes me an individual person is not some essential quality or characteristic, not even a name, but the continued *evolution* of my identity, which takes on different meanings in various settings and in different functions. One can hardly overestimate the consequences of this reorientation from an earlier conceit of static identity. The essentiality of change has pervasively affected how we construct our world and how we build our very identities.

Nietzsche's thought remained deeply connected with the overarching Darwinian tradition from which it received inspiration. At the same time, Nietzsche steadfastly held onto the notion of the autonomous self, and it is at this interesting intersection, where both indeterminancy and autonomy reign, that Nietzsche's influence is so keenly appreciated. Holding these opposing ideas together in an uncomfortable tandem, he reflects our own quandary. We indeed regard ourselves as Selves, but we are hard pressed to say what that in fact means. So as we now turn more specifically to Nietzsche's influence on our notions of health and illness, it is well to remember that his commitment to a Self, albeit a multiperspectival, adaptive, dynamic, and thus elusive self, still serves as the core of his idea of organism.

In both his biological and moral constructions of the self, Nietzsche stands at the source of a philosophy which may be fairly regarded as the extreme modernist position of selfhood. He served as a central architect of the "self-centered solution," and we are the beneficiaries of his achievement in turning the problem of an escaped essence into the very basis of the self's definition. His argument begins with an understanding of Darwinism that is extrapolated to a philosophy of the body. Nietzsche conceived of the body as a dynamic system emerging from favorable internal (and often unrecognized) struggle and competition. He took the struggle between species, the popular understanding of Darwinian evolution of the time, and internalized it, applying the struggle to the individual organism. Thus for Nietzsche, the body was composed of competing "drives" or instincts that vied for hegemony; the stronger drives survived, and in their contest, the domineering drives would continue to war against persistent challenges. This, he thought, was not only a fundamental characteristic of organic processes, but also of the very health of the organism. Thus, in Nietzsche's view, health is not only the capacity of the body through its drives to overcome resistance, but its willingness to pose such resistance as well.

Thus the self expressed its "will to power" through the body. As opposed to "consciousness" or the "soul" which had preoccupied earlier metaphysicians, Nietzsche's biological formulation was the foundation of his thought. The primary and essential characteristic of being human, he held, was to be aware of the body. He criticized Judeao-Christian morality precisely because as these religions denied the body's primacy, so too they denied our essential biological nature. He was fundamentally concerned both to reduce the exalted human to the animal, physiological level of the organic, and to philosophically explicate the status of the body as such. The "will to power" or the various "drives," steered by individual wills to power, constructs the human being as an intraorganismically struggling, multiplicitous, hierarchical body.

The challenge Nietzsche bequeathed us is not that the self is contingent, but rather that it is elusive. More to the point, he charged that no "norm" defines selfhood, but rather that the self *defines itself* as it strives toward some undeclared and nebulous ideal. There is no "normal"—for that would presuppose a pre-Darwinian notion of stable and definable boundaries. The self evolves. The self is not a given, but lives dynamically and dialectically, evolving through time—developmentally and experientially. Its boundaries ever-changing, the self is constantly in the process of redefinition. Evolution without direction or goal—like history without teleology—is evolution *sui generis*, a *value* in itself. Man gropes toward the ideal, but this ideality is not definable.

Much commends Nietzsche's formulation. It resonates with both our romantic tradition and our political commitment to individualism. But there is a darker side to his philosophy: the isolation of the moral agent.

The individual succeeds only to the degree that he asserts his autonomy: an ethics based on consideration for another is left moot. The lingering fault with an autonomy-based ethics is perhaps exemplified by this Nietzschean disregard for others. In the preoccupation with the self-contained self, the positive ethic of self-responsibility and self-realization can easily tip over into "selfishness," "autocracy," and self-consuming narcissism. When so perverted, innervated energy converts to power as domination. Nietzsche the cultural physician versus Nietzsche the proto-fascist continues to generate debate. I am sensitive to the political consequences of his thought and how easily his portrait of humankind suited the Nazi racists. Irrespective of his own disavowal of racism, Nietzsche's philosophy has served as a pedestal for the worst forms of political ideology stretching from German fascistic extreme to American libertarian thought. We need not travel that road in this discussion, however. Suffice it to note that Nietzsche's philosophy may well falter on the the problem of human relationship.

Why cannot Nietzsche satisfactorily account for the Other, and establish the basis of *relation*—a self *with* another? When we dissect the structure of his thought we discern two key elements. The "self-centered" solution has a double meaning: first the *self* is affirmed (albeit with a certain elusive, indefinite quality), but second, the self is in a sense held captive to itself. Nietzsche's philosophy of the self must fail as a basis of a comprehensive ethics, because it eschews the fundamental concern with *intersubjectivity*; it does not realize that after a self is affirmed, it is its relation with others that constitutes the ethical encounter. Nietzsche only carries us part way.

She was beautiful. Young and full of vitality, her auburn hair caught the sun's radiance and struck a halo above clear blue eyes. I recognized her immediately as she approached. I had seen her in the obstetrics clinic the week before. Four months pregnant, she was unwed and alone. In fact, she did not know the father.

Promiscuous, apparently carefree, she had no doubts of her own volup-tuousness. Bountiful breasts and a jaunty walk drew attention to her from women and men alike. I was self-conscious as she beckoned to me. Quickly crossing the street, she greeted me nonchalantly.

"Hi! Do you remember me?"

"Of course. How have you been?"

"Okay. No problems. Hey, do you have time for a cup of coffee? I live only a few blocks from here."

"Well, that would be nice, but I have some things to do. You know, being a medical student is busy."

"Oh come on," she smiled, "I'll make it worth your while. I like you . . . a lot."

I felt myself flush, suddenly caught in the gravitational pull of her beauty. "Oh. Thanks." She stood there before me in all her golden availability. Ripe. Lambent. Ready. My patient.

"Thanks, but I have to run." Pause. "Really." Pause. Then, "Be sure to take your iron!" We parted and deliberately I would not look back.

Even after all these years, I still catch myself wondering about her.

Changes, adjustment, improvement are the responses of life to its challenges, both external and from within. The ideal, the possible, the elusive potential has replaced our sense of the finitude of a bounded world. Awash in this uncertain cosmos is the self, whose own sense gathers tenuously within elusive boundaries and a pliable structure. In this sense, Nietzsche is the author of postmodern Man. Our shifting boundaries make us uncomfortable. We seek definition within a modernist tradition, as did Nietzsche. Scholars debate whether he is the last modern or the first postmodern, the culmination of one tradition or the beginning of another. He is of course both, as are we. The striving for freedom as self-aggrandizement is clearly articulated by Nietzsche the modernist, whose ideals still allow for autonomy and self-actualization; as elusive as such an identity might be, it still seems to represent an attainable ideal. Yet we remain with no firm construct by which to structure that project.

But to examine his thesis is useful for it resonates with so much in our collective psyche about what it is to be human. American history and current culture celebrate the individual who aspires to attain his or her full potential, whether measured in social status, financial wealth, or any other realization. Perhaps more dramatically than any other writer, Nietzsche has captured the primacy of our struggle as autonomous individuals to pursue our own goals. To do so we must act as selves. But at the same time, he has also demonstrated the provisionality of our selfhood. Not only may we *aspire* to change, but we do change, evolving personally, whether we will or not. He thus delineates the issues pertinent to defining selfhood in our postmodern world, where the challenge of ever-changing identity, conditional on cultural values and historical necessity, leaves a subject *qua* ethical agent disturbingly undefined. Beyond our own desires, what guides us in our attempts to live a moral life?

From Locke's politically autonomous legal citizen to Nietzsche's self-contained moral agent, the challenge we are left with is how to place such an individual back into the social world, where encounter constitutes our very being as selves. My overarching strategy is to erect a scaffold between the "self" and the "other" on which to build an ethical edifice: The *self* serves as one end of a figurative pole, and the *other*, the opposite end. They are related by this bridge but more deeply, to borrow an image from physics, they can exist only as a dipole—to have one is to have the other. So, what at first glance appears as two independent elements I will construe as a dipole, a single whole: self and other must, and can, only exist linked. One question is how; I will argue that the *other* serves a constitutive role in defining the *self*. This is germane to our project of delineating an ethics that is responsive to medicine's relational structure. I will suggest that we look elsewhere for guidance, but first let me glean another critical element from Nietzsche's thought.

Health as an Ideal

Nietzsche's philosophy is interesting in its own right, at the very least as it develops the notion of self from its Lockean origins. But we have another agenda, one that directly relates to our inquiry concerning medical ethics. Nietzsche offered us a specific application of his philosophy to the issues of health and disease, and it is here that we must dig a bit deeper to find even stronger supports for our own platform. Having considered Nietzsche's philosophy of body, we can now turn to his notions of health, which gradually evolved to dominate his worldview and would ultimately serve his new morality. To read Nietzsche, one need not extrapolate his thinking to a medical scenario, for his philosophy is clearly informed by his own clinical experience as patient. Throughout his writings, one is struck with Nietzsche's exquisite delineation of what it means to be sick and how it is possible to heal. After all, few modern philosophers have been so preoccupied with their bodies. For Nietzsche—wracked by suffering with both pathological medical and psychosomatic illnesses—health and disease dominated much of everyday existence and served as prominent personal concerns. This biographical fact might be relevant to those psycho-historical "explanations" of his philosophy that many have offered, but I bring it up here rather to attend to Nietzsche's construction of the Self as elusive and changing, and to the implications of that insight.

Although Nietzsche changed his views over time, adding elements and eliminating others, a consistent reading of "health" does emerge. We might characterize this in the following way: (1) Life is defined by struggle and disharmony at all levels; the ability to harmonize and create order from chaos is a measure of individual power; (2) absent absolute truth, God, and absolute good and evil, one can only live well, seeking those values most conducive to powerful, self-creative life; resultant activities may range from aesthetic creation to warlike conquest in the name of such values; (3) since self-creation involves constant redefinition in a changing environment, one must constantly pose resistances to oneself and overcome them. Inability even to muster such resistance represents sickliness; inability to overcome such resistance reveals sickness; and ability both to pose and overcome such resistance represents health—great health; (4) since each individual is the outcome of a unique, contingent history of struggle, and since greatness can be accomplished in many ways, no two types of individual greatness need be equal; hence, there is no single static norm of health—the only constant of health is the degree of power that individuals expend successfully; (5) health of the body and health of the mind are not only physiologically related, but operate according to parallel principles of resistance, struggle, and creative overcoming. Therefore, the great thinker is healthy when he can challenge his principles and incorporate anomalies into new and expanded worldviews.

For Nietzsche, then, health manifests the active search of the "will to power" as it overcomes resistances in a constant process of redefinition. Health is the will to seek resistance and to overcome; it is a measure of the will to power, if any such measure exists. Will is the active, not reactive, self. On this formulation, health as a reflection of the life of the individual shows Nietzsche to be the anti-nihilistic physician of the soul, and finally, the physician of culture. The prescribed ethic becomes a self-centered effort by which we jolt the thoughtless inertia of our lives into a constant self-critique that directs its energies toward a self-defining ideal. In this sense, Nietzsche's thought is thoroughly permeated by an evolutionary metaphysics. Change is of the essence, but it must be harnessed to a self-fulfilling goal. The ethic is thus not only based on the realization that change is an essential component of our being—it is transfigured into a drive toward self-perfection.

Nietzsche's disjointed writings, aphoristic style, and poetic hyperbole notwithstanding, a consistency of purpose and direction defines his thought. He endeavored to become physician to the soul, presenting a means to achieving a transvaluation of values, an ethos of self-realization and growth. His elucidation of the exuberance of the will to power is firmly anchored in a characterization of the organic that is guided by a normative psychological ideal to "become." And overarching the entire enterprise is the autonomy of the individual, a strengthening of the Lockean project in ways that the Englishman would hardly have recognized. We live with the strengths and liabilities of that formulation.

Nietzsche essentially cured his own negative nihilism by affirming continual and creative self-overcoming and self-perfection; this was a philosophy of ideality and self-responsibility. Sickness becomes a metaphor for our diseased times, a cultural extrapolation from our biological natures; health, in turn, is a metaphor for our ethical response. Hence, the philosopher as physician of soul and culture challenges prevailing principles by forcing society and its individuals to acknowledge and incorporate anomalies in their own *Weltanschauung*.

This formulation serves as Nietzsche's foundational conception of health, and it resonates richly with our cultural experience of disease. I suspect that many of our wide-spread notions of health reflect these same commitments to self-responsibility—the struggle each of us must make to attain health—and the powerful stigma we attach to sickness or disability. Susan Sontag, in *Illness as Metaphor*, describes how tuberculosis in the nineteenth century and cancer in our own time have been regarded almost universally as evil, invincible predators, not just diseases of organic misadventure. Illness becomes a metaphor for corrupted souls, serving as intimate reflections of our moral imperfections and weaknesses.

Disease is what speaks through the body, a language for dramatizing the mental: a form of self-expression. . . . Illness reveals desires of which the patient probably was unaware. Diseases—and patients—become subjects for decipherment. And these hidden passions are now considered a source of illness. (pp. 43–44)

More profoundly, disease often serves as a metaphor for our moral predicament. Against environmental pollutants, the price of our decadent technicological society, Nature takes her revenge in the form of cancer; with AIDS, nature is said by some to punish deviant sexual practice.

So, following the close connection we tend to make between infirmity and personal weakness is the perceived punitive nature of disease: we often feel that our illness is our punishment for misdeeds. This attitude is amply illustrated in typical reactions to patients with AIDS. The image of a plague was quickly assigned to the spread of HIV, and as Sontag noted in *AIDS and Its Metaphors*, plagues are invariably regarded as judgments on society.

The basic confusion of seeing illness as metaphoric for the corruption of our very selves again resides in the conception of identity, specifically, in just how the person and his or her disease are identified. If we do not distinguish patient and disease and then go on to evaluate the morality of the homosexual community, then we can easily conflate the illness of the afflicted. As Max Navarre poignantly wrote in "Fighting the Victim Label,"

As a person with AIDS, I can attest to the sense of diminishment at seeing and hearing myself constantly referred to as an AIDS victim, an AIDS sufferer, an AIDS case—as anything but what I am, a person with AIDS. I am a person with a condition. I am not that condition.

If, on the other hand, we recognize person and disease to be separate categories, we will not conflate them and morally castigate, if not condemn the individual who has become ill.

Sexually transmitted diseases traditionally have been used as a tool for stigmatization, where identification and punishment of a transgressing group serve to ostracize those with the disease as outsiders from the culture at large. Irrespective of the travesty of such an assignment, our recent experience with AIDS again shows how the experience of illness draws upon a primitive identification: disease used metaphorically as a window into the person and his or her moral standing. The particularities of AIDS offer us a vivid illustration of an extreme case, which exemplifies our general orientation toward disease and helps us better comprehend the experience of illness as a fundamental manifestation of personal failure. This attitude is well articulated by Nietzsche, who also captured the moral dimension of being sick as the sign of weakness, the sign of an impoverished will.

The autonomous self, then, in serving as the vehicle for responsibility, assumes both a positive empowerment, when viewed in terms of political rights, and a negative one, in the context of pejorative self-debasement where disease is regarded as judgment. The latter is, of course, an ancient sentiment. Consider Jesus addressing the paralytic as he cures him: "My son, your sins are forgiven" (Mark 2:5). Having expressed faith, the paralytic is rewarded; unsaid, but implied, is that he was afflicted for his transgressions. But this pervasive idea of illness as stigma carries two very different moral messages, depending on whether we conceive of the individual within an autonomy-based or a communal-based morality. In the former, the stress is on self-responsibility for cure, because autonomy-based moral systems emphasize the freedom of, and hence responsibility for, action and choice. On the other hand, on an ethic that emphasizes the communality of the individual, the focus is on reciprocity of care. The body politic as a whole must cooperate to bring the patient back into the fold. Curing is caring, and the community, as opposed to the individual, assumes that responsibility.

Beyond the protection of individual rights, the issue of autonomy in medicine has the added dimension of isolation. Autonomy in fact separates the individual from the community and in the setting of illness, the autonomous patient becomes situated on a complex continuum stretching from independence to loneliness. Some may thrive on such an ethic; but in my experience most do not, for their power of individuation has been severely compromised by sickness. In this sense, to suffer is to be alone, adrift in a sea of confusion and isolated by forces beyond one's comprehension and control. The most primitive experience of disease is precisely this very loss of autonomy, of self. I believe the patient is poorly served by such an ethic. We must search elsewhere for an alternative ethics for medicine.

"Doc, I need to talk with you."

"Sure, Mr. Jackson. What's on your mind?"

"I'm a little embarrassed, but you know . . . my wife's cancer . . . well . . ."

"Go ahead Mr. Jackson, what's wrong?"

"Well, do you think that God punishes sin?"

"It's not important what I think. . . . what do you believe?"

"Well, I do, and I think God is punishing me for being untrue."

"To whom?"

"Unfaithful to my wife."

"What are you saying?"

"Well, I'm trying to say that I've been with another woman, and God is punishing me by giving my Cynthia cancer."

We talked about his guilt, but Mr. Jackson's theology was so different from my own that I made no headway in relieving him of his burden. The discussion ended with his declaring, "Thanks Doc, but all I can do now is pray that God will forgive me. I'll be good and maybe Cynthia will recover."

But I knew the response Mr. Jackson would receive from his God. At age 34, Cynthia had metastatic ovarian carcinoma. She would leave two young children bereft of their mother within the year.

3

The Breakdown of Autonomy

The Romantic Reaction and the Aftermath

He was about 30 years old, balding, thin, with a doughy, pale complexion, and in no obvious distress. Sitting placidly on the examination table, in a johnny, his filthy clothes and muddied shoes were piled on the floor. He had told the nurse that he wanted to be evaluated for a rash. I came in and sat down. Looking at the walk-in clinic fact sheet, I saw he listed no address. "So, Mr. Anderson, where are you living?"

"A shanty, surrounded by brush. To call the dwelling a shanty is to give exaggerated structure to the flimsy support poles and patchwork cardboard, canvas, wood and cloth remnants constituting its walls and roof. It is buttressed against the foundation of the expressway and is partially protected and further assimilated by a grove of young saplings and bushes. The shanty does have an aesthetic quality with a careful mixture of Bedouin blue, a lilac, amber and rose sprinkled between the nondescript grays and browns. I quite like it."

I looked at him blankly. Obviously taken aback, I managed to ask him, "Um, yes, and what do you do?"

"I play the tambourine."

"You what?!"

"Tam! tamarin, tamale, tame, tamarack, tambour, tampon, tamarisk, tampion, tamboura . . . tambourine!"

Choosing to ignore this short outburst, I calmly observed, "You look a bit thin. Have you been eating regularly?"

"Food . . . let me think—ah, 'ood.' Yes ood. If I was a boustrophedon!"
Laughing and bending down, with his back to me and sticking his head
between his legs, he rapidly recited, "Poo, poor, poon, poodle, and Pooh!
At Pooh's Corner, that is where we are!"

He straightened up and almost wearily got back on the table, stretched
out on his back and slowly pulled up the front of the johnny; I assumed
he was about to show me his rash. There, where his genitalia were supposed
to be, was a little stub.

"I cut them off . . . three years ago."

I looked, dumbfounded. He smiled wanly and then rolled over to exhibit
the flaming redness between his buttocks, caked with dried feces.

"Wait here, I'll get you some ointment." I rushed out of the room.

Well before Nietzsche, thinking of the fixed, "punctual" self as a fiction
initiated a major metamorphosis of our sense of personal identity. This
transition traces back to the Romantic period, when various cultural and
historical forces converged to celebrate the self in a novel fashion. In many
respects our modern conception of man dates to this period at the end of
the eighteenth century. When Johann Wolfgang von Goethe (1749–1832)
left Weimar to journey to Italy and Samuel Taylor Coleridge (1772–1834)
hiked with his friend William Wordsworth (1770–1850) through the hills
of England, their poetic quests were more than aesthetic excursions. They
sought to redefine themselves in the broadest context of their natural setting. The roots of our contemporary environmentalism grew from this
period, and the urgency of protecting nature is driven by the sentiment
that our own true selves are best situated there. On this view, the city is
corrupting, and we must commune with nature to recapture our better
selves. This projection into the cosmos of our individual psyches is a basic
Romantic notion, and it represents a dethroning of rationality's dominance
and its replacement by a more comprehensive participation in the world.
To achieve such an integration, the boundaries of the self were first loosened and then set free altogether.

The Romantic expressive psyche was expansive, even plastic to the contours of nature and the self-reflexive process of awakening to its glory.
Deliberately and self-consciously, men and women of this time sought to

refashion their identities by exploring nature, both human and nonhuman, to establish new contours of their souls. They sought rapturous insight and aesthetic pleasure. Their spirituality moved beyond a narrow theistic consciousness to a pantheism encompassing the full range of human experience. Rationality would not restrict their journeys, nor would conventional notions of socially prescribed achievement. These romantic wanderers reached beyond themselves (as defined by an Enlightenment rational ideal) to novel personae ruled by the primacy of subjectivity and emotional fulfillment.

The key element in the Romantic journey was a self that was neither rigidly restricted by social convention nor confined to a particular rationality. The expressive self, fluidly dispersed, would revel in the world's splendor and thereby enrich its own experience. Fulfillment was found not in preserving identity but in expanding it. It is no coincidence that Coleridge took mind-altering opiates and like Daedelus sought to reach the sun. The self, no longer set, established, or structured, was now an organic *process* of experience. In loosening the self-contained (and self-sufficent) nature of personhood, the Romantic self became largely defined in relation to its object. That object could be the outside world or some inner reality. Relation became the key precept, for when we are in dialogue, communion, or rapture, the experiencing self is absorbing and responding. In the process of experience, the watchword of Romanticism, the very idea of a set identity, one fixed and unchanging (and thus incapable of response) becomes anathema. The cardinal rule is self-reflection, and in an endlessly recursive process, the self experiences itself, more particularly its world, the other, and its own experience. *Relation* has replaced entity.

In philosophy, the Romantic poets had their counterpart in Georg Wilhelm Friedrich Hegel (1770–1831) and those who reacted to him, the most famous of whom were Karl Marx (1818–1883) and Søren Kierkegaard (1813–1855). Hegel made dialectical thinking central to his philosophy. The basic structure of his thought is that in the meeting of two forces or entities, an integration or synthesis occurs that gives rise to another force or entity, distinguished from the first two in their novel combination. This synthetic product then goes on to have its own encounters; and, endlessly, the world evolves by such dialectical processes. Dialectics may be understood as the simple combination of two elements, say hydrogen and oxygen, to form a new substance, water. Another example is that of two companies merging to form a new corporation that goes on to undertake different enterprises. Hegel applied this basic concept to history, culture, and the self. On this view, the subject relates only to that which it constructs or confronts. In that meeting the realization of the self is determined in a complex duality: the encountered world comprising one element of the synthesis, and the person's own self-consciousness the other. Thus the Self depends intimately on its relation to the "Other," whether God, nature, culture, history, or other selves. Otherness becomes constitutive of self—quite a different vision from that of Kant, in which the self retained individuality and autonomy.

Alterity, the philosophical term for "otherness," revolves around whether and how, in response to an encounter, the self articulates itself or is altered as a consequence of that engagement. How might the engaged self alter its object and their shared world? How might the self live in its world and in a universe of other selves? The self alone is either isolated, hence alienated, or else it actively engages the world, and thereby becomes actualized. This was the basis of Marx's economic theory of self-alienating work and Kierkegaard's religious philosophy of dialogue with the divine, in which, the self's authenticity resides in its responsiveness to that call. *Relation,* whether to work (Marx) or to God (Kierkegaard), was seen in a new light, as the dialectical structure of Hegel's philosophy was taken in new directions. The continued application of this construction to moral, religious, and political philosophies can hardly be overemphasized.

The relational construct as applied to the specific issue of personhood converges on how the potential for self-aggrandizement must be realized *in* the world, and the self must ultimately actualize itself in the encounter with the other. The Other includes the Self—herein lies the essential mystery of our notions of selfhood. This conclusion arises from a radical formulation which has yet to become fully established in our general culture: We are self-consciously aware of our selfhood as arising from our thinking about being a self; but there is a critical caveat—*the self thereby dissolves.* We become locked into a relentless recursive reflection where the self no longer abides as a circumscribed, self-contained entity, "punctual" or otherwise. The self has become immersed in its world, and when one attempts to arrest that experiencing subject by reflecting on its experience, we lose our own subjectivity and substitute an alien objectivity that is fundamentally incapable of capturing what we intuitively refer to as our inner identity, the experiencing self. In short, as soon as we seek to identify our personhood, it slips away into its own recesses.

And from the point of view of moral philosophy, alterity assumes another dimension. Traditionally, the concept of otherness emphasized our responsibilities toward others, in a community as governed by a given moral law. Of course, one example of such communities, namely, those based in adherence to a divinely inspired moral code, long predates the Romantic reaction of the nineteenth century that asserted the primacy of the expressive self, the assertion of self-will and the ethical essentiality of the autonomous moral agent. In many ways, the declaration of the Self, the free spirit, the actualizing individual which characterized the age of Byron, Keats, and Shelley, remains the source of our preoccupation with autonomy in an expressive sense. But the Romantic preoccupation with the psychological independence of the individual also inherited the Enlightenment's tradition of relegating self-responsibility and freedom to a self-governing ethical agent. In short, there are competing claims for the self—one of independence and one of responsibility; one based on autonomy, the other on relation. With Nietzsche's declaration that "God is dead," we witness the ultimate proprietorship of our actions—both as private individuals and public citizens. The crucial twist was the herald of an autonomous *self-defining* ethical being. The self-referential nature of Nietzsche's Self was a debt paid to the Romantics, and so we witness the see-saw nature of the philosophical discourse.

In the 1880s, at the same time that Nietzsche wrote his major works, William James (1842–1910) was wrestling with the issue of selfhood, more specifically, with the elusive nature of such an entity. James was a highly complex personality. Trained as a physiologist, he endured debilitating depression and emerged to study psychology, which evolved to a commitment to philosophy. He became our premier *fin de siècle* philosopher, not only for popularizing pragmatism, that quintessential philosophical product of American culture, but also for delineating the contours of mind and personal identity that resonated with his time, and our own. Heavily influenced by Ralph Waldo Emerson (1803–1882) and the particular New England expression of Romanticism, transcendentalism, James epitomized the intellectual's self-awareness of the limits of rationality and the legitimacy of subjectivity.

As a psychologist and philosopher of mind, James was concerned with exploring the question of personal identity by probing the nature of consciousness (still very much on the agenda of contemporary philosophy). In *The Principles of Psychology*, discussing consciousness, James clearly articulated the elusiveness of mind, and thus of self: "[I]t [consciousness] is not one of the *things experienced* at the moment; this knowing is not immediately *known*. It is only known in subsequent reflection." According to James, consciousness can only be regarded as a process, in whose attempt to objectify experience, that is to share it and make it public, consciousness is transformed into something else altogether. Our reflection on our thought, on our perception, on our feelings, is irretrievably distinct from the source of that process that we would like to refer to as our inner or core self. The act of recognition is itself a function of our self-awareness, and as consciousness or actions are reviewed, a continual generation of new experience must in turn be contemplated. The act of introspection is thus perpetually incomplete in the attempt to capture the primary experience. The reflection itself is a thought—and then the recursive spiral begins and there is no end. James came upon a deep insight: The self (and by now I hope the metaphor has dissuaded any attempt at concretization) is truly unaware of itself as it acts. In our actions we *are*, and any contemplation of such behavior can only be relegated to the same collective—mental forms of persons acting in the world.

The psychological elusiveness of selfhood elicits a beguiling puzzlement. There is no ready definition of the self outside specific contexts, independent of particular languages and social or physical settings. For instance, selves as citizens have certain rights and obligations as defined by law; men or women as basketball players are defined by the rules of the game and their performances; soldiers as selves are defined by their military roles and duties; patients are defined by their pathologies and reports of illness. So when we speak of the self, we are actually only referring to a commonly accepted construction, one formed out of the contingency of a particular time and place. The self has become a convenient vehicle for speaking about various social roles. When extended to our personhood, the concept becomes a conundrum.

Postmodernism and the Self

I went in search of myself.
Heraclitus, XXVIII

Our discussion of the identity of self can now be brought under the general heading of "postmodernism." Arnold Toynbee, the British historian, used the term to signify the end of an era marked by Western domination. In this latter sense, postmodernism referred to the last phase of Western history, an era supposedly marked by irrationalism, anxiety, and lost hopes. Notoriously difficult to define, postmodernism has assumed many other connotations as it has been applied to art, literature, film, architecture, political theory, philosophy, psychology, sociology, science, and religion. Our concern here is of the general understanding of the self as adopted by this point of view. I will sketch it briefly.

In many respects, postmodernism may be regarded as a continuation of the Romantic reaction to the Enlightenment. We have yet to complete the deconstruction of the self that began in the early nineteenth century. The Romantics had no intention of eliminating the idea of selfhood; but in their initiating its expansion, the concept of identity began to lose its boundaries. Eventually the very question of an entity that we might designate "the Self" became highly problematic. Post–World War II literary, artistic, and philosophical expression has focused upon the logical extension of the problem, often characterized as that of the self's indeterminacy. I use "indeterminacy" in the sense currently fashionable in literary criticism, that texts have no single correct interpretation, and not only because readers may differ in their respective understandings, but more profoundly, because language itself has no restraints on its reference. Since there is no fixed point within or without the text, meanings proliferate and change with viewpoint and with time, and the meaning of the text as a whole is indeterminate. Applied to our consideration of the self, indeterminacy provides a revolutionary perspective.

I think such deconstructive critiques resonate deeply with the problem of identity. Specifically, I refer to the centrality of the Self in relation to the Other as a radical expression of post-structuralism, a particular character in postmodern thought. Structuralism understands meaning to be a function of the relations among the components of any cultural formation, or of our very consciousness. For instance, the pictures of the mind's world assume their meaning, value, and significance from their relationships—that is their "place" within a structure. But the post-structuralists broadly argued that any structure crumbles when we recognize that no part can assume participation outside its relation to other parts. In other words, there is no center, no organizing principle privileged over structure that would thus be able to dominate its structural domain. From this perspective, there is nothing natural about cultural structures (e.g., language, kinship systems, social and economic hierarchies, sexual norms, religious beliefs), no transcendental significance to limit "meanings," and only power explains the hegemony of one view over another. Similarly, the Self may be regarded as constructed by arbitrary criteria, so that it occupies no natural habitat. This scenario radically challenges the insistence on the Self's dependence on the Other: Not only has the Self's autonomy been rendered meaningless, *any* construction of the Self is regarded as arbitrary.

The common element with the postmodernist view of selfhood is that the Self, like the rest of the world, has no reference point, and must be regarded as having melted away. As C. S. Lewis (1898–1963) quipped, "the Subject is as empty as the Object." When the subject is "decentered," no longer an origin or a source, it becomes the merely contingent result or product of multiple social and psychological forces. On this view, the unity of the Self is at best a deceptive construct. Its very authenticity has been fundamentally challenged. In short, from this perspective, the Self should more appropriately be viewed as a contingency, or an interpretive scheme. If the Self is a contingency, there is no unity by which it may be organized to confront its world. The postmodern view of the Self disallows Kant's modern subject to determine for itself, completely and unconditionally, what to accept as evidence about the nature of its world, or its organization. Self-determination has been replaced by some choice, for better or for worse; a construction based on the unsteady assumptions of cultural practice and historical chance.

Another critical assault on the idea of the Self rose from the philosophy of Ludwig Wittgenstein (1889–1951). Arguably, of twentieth-century analytical philosophers, Wittgenstein became the major arbiter of philosophy's limits. As a philosopher of mathematics, logic, and language, he was to radically critique these fields, leaving us with major uncertainties concerning the logical basis by which we might understand ordinary language. He bequeathed a tradition of analysis that restricts the province of logic to logic, of knowledge to science, and of ethics to the metaphysical, where philosophy's analytical tools were inapplicable in each case. His message was that we are on tenuous ground when we try to assess the logical basis of our language, or for that matter when we try to understand our very thought (for language and thought are inseparable). Philosophy's role, then, was to "show the fly out of the bottle," or in other words, to demonstrate our faulty thinking when we believe we have finalized a philosophical problem. And the Self was such a problem.

Wittgenstein had precious little to say explicitly about the Self. In his notebooks, written in World War I trenches and military prison camps, he sighs about the Self as "deeply mysterious." Consequently scholars have actively debated Wittgenstein's position. A distillation of the discussion yields two primary concepts: Wittgenstein's views are severely solipsistic. In a fundamental sense, only the Self exists; the world exists for the Self; thus is "knowledge" achieved. And second (therefore), it is nonsense to even attempt to define such a Self, since there is no external Archimedean point by which a knowing entity might survey or characterize itself other than in the totality of its experience: We cannot see ourselves from the outside. Because of the lack of coordinates for any discussion of these matters, Wittgenstein declined to muse about such a metaphysical construction as selfhood. But in his later philosophy he offered a possible vehicle for at least understanding the appeal that such a construct might hold for us. The Self, Wittgenstein would have argued if pressed, only "exists" as part of a "language game," a convention within which it possesses some explanatory value. But to define that value is a seemingly hopeless task, and more importantly, a vacuous one. Neither logic nor science can establish a basis for defining the Self, and any attempt to do so sinks into the ambiguities of other metaphysical constructs, such as "mind." We might want to discuss consciousness, but we can only examine neurological function, measure brain electrical activity, trace nerve networks, assess biochemical transmitters. We *are*, and that is that.

James's influence here is obvious, and clearly Wittgenstein read James carefully and with respect. Wittgenstein's profoundly disturbing philosophical critique radically extended what, in the 1890s, seemed to represent a sophisticated psychological description. In Wittgenstein's hands, the Self, which had been so influential in forming our post-analytic philosophy, is no longer decentered—it has vanished altogether. Selfhood is rendered a meaningless metaphysical construct that cannot be analyzed or concretized in any fashion. To try to do so is to speak nonsense. We obviously do speak of "the self," but this is an expression in our language game, a particular social convenience that allows us to communicate—it has no logical or scientific basis. As a category of knowledge, the Self has dissolved, a discarded remnant of an older metaphysics.

This is the extreme radicalism of a post-philosophical analysis. Beyond the Self as a relational construction or a decentered subject defined by contingent cultural constructions, *the Self as an entity simply does not exist.* If this position is taken seriously, the basis of an ethics evidently dissolves. Who is the moral agent, and how is he or she defined? How can we ask about responsibility *if we cannot even define the moral agent?* Wittgenstein's fascinating, nihilistic response: Ethics is known, morality is enacted, but to require a philosophical answer as to how and why is to give false answers and to invoke deceptive rationalities, distorted by prejudice and only supposedly buttressed by logical argument. Ethics derives from beyond rationality; its ground is metaphysical. And, said Wittgenstein, metaphysics cannot be analyzed.

On this view, philosophy's role in this post-analytic era is to discern what is amenable to philosophical analysis (largely a technical endeavor) and what is not. If one is a Wittgensteinian, philosophy is unable to address many of its traditional questions. Its primary role is to disenchant us from thinking that we are being "philosophical" in the sense of offering logical or analytical "solutions." The narratives we weave around the classic philosophical issues such as personal identity are simply delusional, if we expect some kind of logical formulation of the problem. In Wittgenstein's terminology, questions of this kind are "nonsense" because they are bereft of final adjudication. In contrast, such a question as "Is it raining?" demands a meaningful response: "Yes, it is raining" or "No, it is not raining." So for Wittgenstein, only certain questions were "meaningful," and he turned to science as a paragon of such inquiry. Scientists deal with meaningful questions, because the answers investigators glean from nature can be verified by objective means. But discussions regarding the Self can offer no such knowledge. Instead, we speak in generalities that may easily be disputed, depending on the perspective adopted or the evidence that one chooses to bring to the debate. Although discussions about the Self may be important, we must recognize their true character: perhaps holding relevance and revealing erudition within religious, literary, psychoanalytic, political, ideological, or historical contexts, such debates should never be confused as philosophical, thus meaningful in Wittgenstein's sense.

This conclusion leaves us in a quandary. Our key categories of discussion—the particular topic, medical ethics and the Self—are left in philosophical limbo. I admit to an insecurity in discussing them if we are to adopt Wittgenstein's perspective: The moral domain belongs in the metaphysical beyond, outside such analyses. Ethics may be supported by argument, by analysis, by logic, but no final formulation is possible based on such debates. In other words, from the Wittgensteinian orientation, there is no *philosophical*—that is, analytical—grounding for ethics. And thus there can be no rational or logical structure by which moral questions may be adjudicated as "true" or "false." That is not to say that there is no right and wrong, only that those determinations are made within the moral universe—derived from social, historical, religious discourse—and not the analytical. To discuss morality we might profitably explore traditional philosophical positions, no doubt to great advantage for certain insights, but I would venture another strategy. Let us freely admit the limitations of such analysis and proceed to sketch a metaphysics by which we might tackle our problem. To do so is not to abandon philosophical analysis (after all, metaphysics *was* a branch of philosophy!), but to self-consciously acknowledge those limits and proceed with a different kind of analysis. In other words, I will adopt a postanalytical philosophical stance. And to those who will say that I am engaged in "nonsense," I reply that what we need is an "antiphilosophy." And as we will see, we have one.

Metaphysics?

"Rabbi Cohen died yesterday."

The voice on the telephone was a physician in Israel informing me that my patient and friend, Moses Cohen, had finally succumbed to his malignancy. Cohen was 35 years old and, like me, had a bevy of young children. He was an active politician, a man whose charisma and leadership skills had clearly marked him as a rising star in the firmament of Israeli politics. He had come to my office five years earlier for a consultation. Sitting among the other patients in the waiting room, he had stuck out as an anomaly, a man whose dress and demeanor were distinctly other-worldly. He wore his uniqueness lightly and exhibited no self-consciousness, but it was obvious to all, he at least knew who he was, where he was, and why he was.

His disease was fatal and no therapy would slow its progress. The blood cells grew without control, and as his belly swelled from a huge spleen, other complications arose. He visited me for a second opinion. Israeli doctors were well trained, but a Harvard professor might offer him other options, new hope, a better chance. I assured him that I could not, but he kept returning.

Rabbi Cohen loved to talk, and over the years our discussions often spread beyond the concerns of his disease to his children, his wife, his work. And then, as our intimacy grew, we spoke of religion, of God, of evil. He taught me his religion patiently and with great kindness, and imparted a sense of his faith that not only initiated admiration, but instilled desire for one as powerful as his own. In those encounters our roles reversed and he ministered to my disquiet and confusions. I came to love his compassion, intelligence, verve, and sense of goodness. I was excited whenever I knew he was coming to Boston.

I knew he wasn't doing well. My Israeli colleague had often called for advice, but the suddenness of the announcement left me groping for words. "Thank you for calling. Please convey my condolescences to Esther."

I hung up, stared at the phone, and then lowered my head and wept. I hadn't cried in years.

I suppose it is becoming evident that I am changing my voice from that of a physician to a metaphysician. There is more than wordplay intended here. *Metaphysics* was coined by Aristotle's editor, Andronicus of Rhodes, who placed those books following the *Physics* in a distinctive collection. Hence those writings that simply happened to reside next to Aristotle's scientific writings were designated "metaphysics." If the books had been placed before *Physics* I surmise we would have "prophysics," (before-physics) but we have instead "after-physics," or "metaphysics," following the Greek. Hardly an auspicious beginning for a venerable discipline. But in a sense the definition holds, since metaphysics is generally applied to any inquiry that lies beyond or behind or underneath those questions addressed by science. This is not to say that metaphysics is intrinsically antiscientific—after all, science too has its own metaphysics. Cardinal precepts about reality—its fundamental order and cohesiveness, its knowability through our rational and perceptive faculties, its mathematical harmony and predictability, (or lack thereof in the world of quantum states), and so on—form the metaphysical foundations of physics.

These are some of science's metaphysical claims, which when fully analyzed represent profound philosophical assumptions about thought and its object of inquiry, reality. Philosophers, however, divide between those who consider the metaphysics of science metaphysics enough, and those who go beyond scientific knowledge to apprehend a metaphysical structure of the universe that might be perceived through different kinds of knowledge and experience. This latter group seeks metaphysical principles broader than those of scientific epistemology alone. The question metaphysicians ponder is, How can we present a comprehensive, coherent, and consistent account of reality as a whole? Scientists might fairly claim that this is, in fact, the task they have set for themselves; but a theologian would counter that in overlooking the most important domain of the divine, which cannot be so apprehended, such a metaphysics based solely on scientific knowledge is impoverished and incomplete. But while metaphysics need not be synonymous with theology, in its search for the most persistent and universal characteristics of the cosmos, it becomes the study of ultimate reality, for it is concerned with existence as such, and even more specifically with the assumptions employed by our systems of knowledge in their claims of what is real. By this definition, metaphysics more or less encompasses philosophy, or to be less charitable, is confused with philosophy itself, a fair conflation from Wittgenstein's perspective.

For those seeking some final resolution of the status of metaphysics, philosophy has turned upon itself in a most disturbing way by discovering the limitations of its inquiry. I think it fair to say that it is *philosophically* impossible to achieve the goals of metaphysical inquiry, according to the dominant analytical theory today. This purging of philosophy of what Wittgenstein called the "nonsense" of metaphysical statements (and these included virtually everything outside science) dates at least as far back as David Hume's (1711–1776) quip in the *Enquiry Concerning Human Understanding* that metaphysics should be "committed to the flames, for it can contain nothing but sophistry and illusion." This paragon of the Enlightenment was attacking religion—superstition and bigotry of all sorts—and when regarded as antitheological, the assault on metaphysical thinking has a certain tenacity and validity. Ironically, however, religion's retreat had an unexpected secondary consequence, as philosophy itself came under attack. Following Hume, philosophy has been largely content with the systematic study, not of reality, but the structure of our thought *about* reality.

But the metaphysical impulse survives, and twentieth-century philosophy seems engaged in an endless battle to rid itself of its own metaphysical urges. There have been no dearth of calls to end metaphysics, and we see in such breast-beating the almost poignant self-consciousness—if not the lethal Achilles' heel—of the discipline. In its unflinching self-criticism, philosophy must remain committed to the sanctity of its own analysis. And not surprisingly so. After all, the search for universals and the engagement in analysis has an irresistible allure for the philosopher.

As I describe this state of affairs, I know that it is almost impossible to explain to the nonphilosopher what the fuss is all about. But I want to bring this self-conscious attitude to the foreground of our discussion, for my attack on autonomy on the one hand, and my espousal of a relational ethics on the other, are both based ultimately on a frankly metaphysical argument. This means that the basis for my case will borrow freely from a nonanalytical perspective, and in doing so I wish to cut the bonds of those restraints that bind ethics in Wittgenstein's straitjacket. My strategy is to build upon the deconstructive challenges already discussed, where the intersection of the Self at contemporary philosophical crossroads has presented us with an important clue to the nature of how to ground our ethical project. I believe we must employ these postanalytical positions to orient us in approaching how and why medical ethics has stumbled, and furthermore to help us erect a better moral structure for medicine. Let me now return to the specifics of the medical scenario.

Autonomy and Care of the Patient

The pain was intolerable. I had a sudden stab in my back and knew at once that I had a kidney stone. The spasm lasted several minutes, I don't even know how long, but then it ebbed. As I struggled to my feet after writhing in pain on the floor, my son packed me into the car and we drove to the hospital.

There I was efficiently pierced for blood studies and intravenous fluids, and given pain killers. I was in such distress that I could not think. I had no clear idea of what was happening to me. Between the narcotic-induced grogginess and the intermittent agony, I could barely understand my predicament, my options, or the possibility of a resolution.

For over a week I suffered intermittent episodes of pain. I could not pass the stone. Imaging showed the obstruction near my kidney and the bloating of that organ behind the stone. There was no confusion over my condition. Over the next three weeks I continued to have bouts of acute pain, each requiring visits to the emergency room, and once requiring hospitalization. I struggled to decide whether to have surgery or to try to wait out the ordeal. Passing the stone on my own would be best, but increasingly I lost hope in that outcome.

My urologist was almost sanguine in the face of my indecision. Because I was a physician he perhaps was less adamant in his advice, and his counsel was ambiguous. I was to decide, alone. As an adult I had never before this required medical attention. This was my first mature experience as a patient. I was immobilized. I could not make the decision. I kept thinking that maybe one more day was all I needed. I knew the risks of surgery, the postoperative recovery, etc., and still I procrastinated. My doctor left me to anguish and I sought counsel elsewhere, but no one would tell me what to do. They probably didn't take me seriously—the guy who always made decisions couldn't decide whether he was in enough discomfort to have surgery? Silly. They figured if the pain was severe enough I would submit myself to the knife.

Finally, during the sixth pain episode, my urologist made the decision. I was whisked into the operating room.

"Well, Fred, it's time. You've had enough."

I nodded numbly.

In the operating room, before falling asleep, I remember him joking to the anesthesiologist, "This guy is in for an orchidectomy"—in laypersons' terms, a castration. They both laughed and smiled at me as I fell under their spell.

Given the limits of reason and authority, tolerance in a pluralistic society is the foundation of our morality, and we thus return again and again to the Enlightenment's project of liberalism as the basis of medical ethics. But when we frame medical ethics in the context of the commonality of the group in which we all join as individuals, we witness a fascinating tension: Wishing to remain firmly committed to the Lockean ideal of autonomy, we nevertheless have shifted the perspective of concern from the political (or scientifically objective) to the humane, and thus contradictorily subjective, care of a person. The notion of autonomy then must be fitted, as best it can, to other kinds of needs. For autonomous clinical scientists, dispassionate observation and cold logic will hardly suffice in caring for the sufferer. And the patient, in turn, while enjoying his or her rights as an individual, cannot maintain strict autonomy as an independent agent. The fundamental relation between selves has been altered: The patient is no longer an autonomous unit. The patient has become dependent in ways that threaten autonomy at its very core. Beyond attempts to answer the needs of a pluralistic society with the common moral purposes that arise with respect to the individual, medicine must address a different kind of relationship, in which autonomy is only one aspect of a complex calculus of caring. This is the essential basis of defining our ethical behavior as health care providers, a tension that makes the current debates on medical ethics so interesting and important.

In medicine, autonomy is compromised if not fundamentally threatened, albeit for good reason. With modern clinical science, the patient is not only incapable of making a fully informed decision about diagnostic and therapeutic choices; his or her very personhood becomes redefined by illness. For example, suppose I have a pain in my upper back. I go to the clinic for an assessment. While it is my pain, it is also something fundamentally foreign to my personhood. There is a deep disjunction between my pain and my self. This is the first step in the redefinition of my selfness, the separation of my dis-ease from an inner cohesive sense of personhood. This is a crucial step because it allows the segregation of my problem from my self as an autonomous agent. When the sickness is integral to my sense of self, then the clinical balance is shifted from a "clinical problem" to a sick person. Modern medicine does best when focused on the former, and it too often stumbles when a more comprehensive approach is required. Much more will be said on this distinction, but let us first concentrate on the first, simpler case.

The doctor examines me and says the pain seems localized to the eigthth or ninth rib. The ribs are naturally mine, but they are also distinct from me, alien bodies that have taken on an identity somehow separate from me. So as objects of scrutiny, entities somehow separate from my being, I can easily allow their dissection. My doctor pronounces that I need some tests: X-rays, blood tests, perhaps more sophisticated imaging techniques; possibly a biopsy. What are the possibilities? She hems and haws, mentioning a vast array of possible problems, including cancer. CANCER! Good God, not me! I am too healthy and vigorous. I am in the prime of life. I have a family, a job; work to be done; security to attain; responsibilities. My life has hardly begun. Cancer is impossible. But how can I deal with this crisis? Well, the first decision is to put my trust in my doctor. Let her do what is necessary. I trust her. That is the choice . . . and it is my last one. My autonomy has been severely compromised. Certainly I will be given options, consulted about preferences, but in reality she will decide. She will know the context of any result, the alternatives, the priorities. And she will inform me of her best judgment. By acceding to her assessment I have forfeited my autonomy, my ability to choose. Under the circumstances I am more than pleased to relegate this basic component of my personhood to her, allowing my overall individuality to be preserved by her good judgment. Let her deal with this alien body, my ribs, and let her solve my disease.

The physician has attained this authority—in fact, this power—over the patient because she is a scientist. There is an interesting irony here: Science, which as an objective approach to nature and humankind offered a new political ideal in the autonomy of the individual, has, four centuries later, come to threaten the very ideal it helped establish. There are several tributaries to this problem, not the least of which is that science, progressively since Galileo's trial in the early seventeenth century, has undermined the authority of revealed religion, and as a practical consequence has also loosened the hold of transcendent criteria for adjudicating moral behavior. This factor seems to me self-evident. What is less obvious perhaps is how science styles itself upon the same moral structure as its object of scrutiny. Nature *is*; there is no divine influence, no goal, no place for human passions in the scientific assessment. These elements may be introduced later when we contemplate our handiwork, but the scientific act, as it were, is objective. In this sense scientific morality distinguishes itself from theological morality, in which human passion, emotion, and subjectivity play into the calculus of behavior and moral action. In science, none of these personal concerns ostensibly has a role in observing, measuring, or assessing natural phenomena. If anything, the scientific observer should be entirely neutral, if not unseen. Certainly to introduce the scientist's opinion or prejudice into his or her assessment would be tantamount to nullifying this assessment. Modern science at its earliest inception urged a neutral stance for its practitioners, both as they described nature and as they drew their conclusions from those observations.

Although science claimed dispassion and objectivity in observing the universe, an abiding conflict arose when such objectivity became the foundation of medicine. For while we demand a rational and scientific basis for our clinical practice, at the same time we recognize that we require an ethics based on other principles. Where do those principles come from? Most medical ethicists argue by extrapolating from the political world, naming the unalienable rights of autonomous citizens as sufficient to govern an ethical medicine. I disagree, and I do so for three reasons:

• It is obvious that patient autonomy is a conceit. Patients cannot fully exercise autonomy simply for the reason that they lack the training and knowledge to make the complex decisions required today in the setting of a highly technical and obscure clinical science.

• Medicine is fundamentally a parental (some would even say a priestly) function. The care of the patient is based on helping the sufferer, the one who is unable to care for her- or himself. The basic precept of the clinician is to care for the hapless patient, albeit with respect for the individual's autonomy, but essentially driven by the desire to restore that sovereignty which has been lost.

• Science offers a countervailing ethic of dispassion, and thus the aspiration to be objective in dealing with disease cannot address the requisites of a compassionate medicine. (Of course, science is a prerequisite of rational care!) I will maintain that an interpersonal ethics must establish the foundation of medicine as a human praxis and that clinical science serves only as a tool in that endeavor.

These are assertions. I have neither fully illustrated my contentions, nor have I yet argued for an alternative formulation, but the outlines of my concerns have already begun to appear. The political ideal of autonomy is unqualifiedly appropriate in certain settings. In the days of the rugged frontier of North America, survival depended on the ability of individuals to fend for themselves. Popular culture, as well as the reality of conquering a wilderness, enhanced our appreciation of individualism. Autonomy is the judicial and philosophical construction of this political mentality. But there is a countervailing communalism that demands our attention. We live in a complex society where we depend on each other in a fashion hardly imagined by our Enlightenment forefathers. Despite our repeated avowals of a hearty, autonomous citizenry, the reality of community demands a broader sense of the individual.

These issues become quite explicit in medicine, where it is obvious that the doctor-patient relationship is governed by a complex equation of personhood. On the one hand, to suffer or to be in pain is to lose one's full sense of self. We cannot function normally as individuals when we are sick, and thus our ability to be a self is compromised. Medicine must be committed to restoring that integrity, or at least protecting it, when the patient is clearly unable to make any decisions. An important index concerning this matter is the 1991 federal law, *The Patient Self-Determination Act*. This statute mandates that health care institutions provide written information informing patients of their legal rights under state law to make advance directives concerning treatment decisions should they become incompetent. These advance directives are of two types: (1) instructional directives such as living wills and medical directives that detail patient preferences regarding treatment, and (2) proxy designations which establish a power of attorney for health that vest patients' future decision-making rights in specific persons. These directives serve to protect the moral and legal rights of self-determination, diminish uncertainty about what a patient would want done in a medical crisis, and reduce conflict between decision makers over how to administer health care in problematic situations. These goals seem quite appropriate within the political context of autonomy, but critics have raised several interesting problems with the law.

First, the contingency of future self-interests may alter decision choices. These include unanticipated therapeutic options, which might be precluded if the living will overrules the future input of the physician or family. In general, if the preferences are too detailed, the flexibility of choices may become too restricted; by focusing on cessation rather than on continued treatment such mandates will probably not be nuanced enough to fit the patient's future needs. Thus mechanisms that allow overriding advance directives have been discussed that attempt to adhere to the autonomy principle, but in fact skirt it. For instance, one approach assumes the "best interest standard" criterion, which allows the health care proxy powerful decision-making privileges. In this scenario, proxy directives have greater flexibility and more relevance to the patient's actual condition than any prior patient directives possibly could.

The proxy essentially assumes the patient's ability to choose, replacing autonomy with substituted agency. This representative judgment (analogous to representative government vs. direct participatory "town meeting" government) depends on the proxy's ability to discern what the patient would have wanted. But the danger of misinterpretation due to the proxy's projection of his or her own values is always present. This tension may be due to bonafide value differences, or to financial or emotional conflicts of interest. True autonomy requires self-responsibility, and in its dilution we inevitably face such imbroglios. Such is the price of compromise. These matters are highly complicated; we are beginning to see patients executing both instructional and proxy directives, which will likely give rise to conflicts as one set of directives are interpreted differently from the other. Thus the legal rights of the proxy might come to be pitted against the judgment of the physician. Interpreting terms such as "terminal," "futile," "extraordinary," and "artificial means" can become legalistically tortuous as the best interests of the patient are debated in differing contexts.

There is another component to this matter that deserves at least a short discussion: To what extent do patients really *want* autonomy? This is a difficult question to answer, but I was struck recently by a study of patient preferences concerning communication with physicians about end-of-life decisions. In this study, published in 1997 in the *Annals of Internal Medicine* by Jan Hofmann and his colleagues from major medical centers across America, fewer than a quarter of seriously ill people had discussed cardiopulmonary resuscitation with their doctors, and only about ten percent the preference for prolonged assisted ventilation. It was not necessarily that they had no opportunity to do so, for most of them preferred not to deal with these issues at all. Other surveys have shown that concord between physicians' treatments (or family members' directives) and patients' actual wishes is no greater than that dictated by chance. So despite increased public awareness and legislation to address the process by which critical medical decisions are made, we are left with a huge gap in communication between patient and health care provider. The evident reluctance of patients to discuss such questions implies at the least that not all of them necessarily want to make such choices, and we are left with an ideal of autonomy that has substantially less than universal subscription.

The conundrum I have sketched concerning the *Patient Self-Determination Act* revolves around the issue of autonomy, which in the setting of caring for the severely ill becomes an abstraction of questionable utility. So in this context, while we strive to retain autonomy as a persistent ideal that should in some way guide medicine's goals, the ill have undeniably lost their full sense of individuality, and another moral basis must emerge to regulate their care. The terminally ill patient is an extreme case to be sure, but nevertheless he or she remains on the continuum of the paradigmatic doctor- or nurse-patient relationship. In seeking the proper moral code for the entire clinical spectrum, I have described the political and legal ideal of autonomy largely to establish another ethic.

The legal and moral issues concerning the acutely ill patient do not necessarily coincide, and we often witness the divergence of the two in the highly charged setting of the terminally ill. Increasingly, medical ethicists have been regarded as a resource to help sort out problematic cases. In large medical centers they often will be consulted, much as a specialist in infectious diseases or orthopedic surgery is called to help with a problem beyond the expertise of the attending physicians. In this sense, medical ethics may legitimately be regarded as a branch of clinical medicine, having moved from the classroom to the bedside. In light of these demands, it is perhaps not surprising that the discipline has so quickly become a pragmatic, hands-on activity as opposed to a distant, theoretical academic field. But not to explore the deeper philosophical issues at play is to forfeit the opportunity both to direct and to frame our moral options. In the next chapter we turn to an alternative to autonomy-based medical ethics.

4

The Call of the Other

A Calling

"Run and get Mommy my pump."

She was struggling for every breath. Her neck muscles contracting with each inhalation, she spasmodically would shift from arching her back to being hunched over. She would cough and spit, and then issue a long, raucous high-pitched wheeze. I knew the signs of her attacks all too well.

As long as I could remember my mother would have such episodes and I would run around, retrieving various items to aid her struggle. I was expert at pouring liquid bronchodilators into the glass nebulizer inhalation pump, but my duties also extended to the more mundane chores of finding the tissues, filling glasses of water, and rearranging her pillows. At age four I had begun my medical career.

"You are my little man," she would smilingly reassure me. I never was calmed. There was a persistent fear: My mother would die a violent death. I remember an early resolution: I would find a cure for asthma.

I entered medical school in 1969, but my medical education began when I was a small child. My father would take me on his house calls when I was four or five. Given his time commitments, it was our only regular bond, and I watched him closely. I was always impressed by his style. On the rare occasions I actually witnessed him examining a patient, I was struck by his commanding authority. He always dominated the interview. If his patients were well prepared and posed questions on his entry, he would summarily dismiss their complaint or shortly mumble a response.

He was paternalistic, domineering, and at the same time, remote. There was always a certain distance maintained between him and his patient. The working-class men and women whom he served seemed to adore him. The smiling comments they offered when I was introduced always included, "Do you know what a great man your father is?" or "I hope you become a great doctor like your Daddy!" My father thought that his behavior instilled confidence and, more important, respect.

As a physician, the senior Dr. Tauber was a strange combination of aloofness and profound concern. When a patient was doing poorly, he would fret and scurry, visiting her at frequent intervals. If a patient returned with a recurrent tumor, he considered the case a personal failure. When a patient died, he cried, sometimes obsessing for hours over what might have been done to change the course of the illness. He cared deeply. His memory of departed souls evoked a profound sentimentality. Yet with the living he was brusque, and he commandeered them into the most compliant posture. He was happiest when cutting.

Toward the end of high school, my weekends often were highlighted with my joining my father in the operating room for an emergency appendectomy. I would watch in amazement as he would flourish the scalpel, make a darting incision and quickly apply the hemostats. I held the retractors, and peered into the belly. Once I accomplished the art of holding retractors, I learned how to suture the skin. It was great fun.

My father opened an office in 1949 on Good Hope Road, nestled deeply in a blue collar neighborhood. The waiting room was always full, no doubt in part due to his generosity. About one-third of his patients could not afford to pay, and there was no insurance. I remember, each December, stuffing envelopes not with Christmas greetings but year-end bills. He would hand me a pile of matched bills and envelopes, and I was responsible for folding, sealing, and stamping. There was a fair degree of bartering. For instance, my front teeth were broken on an errant swing of a baseball bat and I required root canal work. My father went next door to Gerald Hospas, D.D.S. and begged him to sober up for the operation—professional courtesy and all that. Such courtesies included double parking in front of Mr. Hacker's barber shop and running in for a quick cut, and sometimes a shave. The police never bothered my father; the entire neighborhood obviously respected him.

Then, and even more in the 1960s and '70s, when the "white-coated businessmen" (as my mother referred to his colleagues) were making fortunes from their medical practices, he stood out as almost absentminded about medical finances. He lamented what he perceived to be an undemocratic medical system, advocating socialized medicine as the proper alternative. He thought physicians should be salaried, work in a cooperative group like the Mayo Clinic, and subordinate the financial elements of medical practice to the most important priority, caring for patients. The calling did not include getting rich from the suffering. He would minister to his case, and that was the primary reward. So beneath his brusqueness, his patients and I knew he was truly committed to them. Later, I likened him to Albert Schweitzer, minus the organ and the Bach: condescending to the natives, yet completely committed to their well-being. I suppose my father's example was an important reason that I chose to work in a municipal hospital, where besides the working poor, I cared for the drug addict, the prostitute, the thief.

The early years of medical school were arduous. Medical students yearn for clinical exposure, but there is first the long process of learning medicine's language and adapting to the prescribed professional protocol. Beyond the social apprenticeship lies the sheer enormity of detail to be mastered. Rote memorization was drudgery; I found no conceptual challenge. For me, to learn the sequence of enzymatic steps in the biochemical breakdown of sugars or the insertions of the gluteal muscles into various bones held no *intellectual* interest. I simply learned a new language and was amused by the goings-on of my classmates. Such a heterogeneous bunch. The future psychiatrists huddled together at the back of the room, smirking in their self-satisfaction and supposed intellectual superiority. Those who would be surgeons—no doubt because they comprised a fraternity—made a point of rollicking through that painful period along the lines of *M*A*S*H,* the carefree Don Juans of that elite brotherhood. My friends were the more introspective internists-to-be. We took our studies very seriously, knowing that lives depended on our learning the regulation of thyroid metabolism, the side effects of opiates, the antibacterial spectrum of tetracycline. We were not to be surgeons, or psychiatrists, or radiologists, but *doctors.*

The gravity of my training was punctuated very clearly for me during that first year. I discussed with my father a biochemistry exam. One of the questions involved the use of insulin. My answer had been wrong, and my father's remark sent a chill through my soul: "You would have killed the patient with that therapy." What he made explicit, and what was left largely implicit in our early training, was the awesome *responsibility* of being a doctor. The care of the patient loomed as very earnest business. At our sole discretion, life-or-death decisions would have to be made. More than on intellectual vigor, medical students are also selected on the basis of emotional maturity. Admissions committees rarely err on assessing academic performance; how well unformed youth adapt to the emotional demands of medicine is more difficult to gauge.

Young adults are generally poorly equipped emotionally to handle the gruesome responsibility of caring for the severely ill. They usually have little encounter with suffering, and to witness pain and death, except for a few, has not been part of their intimate experience. Most lead sheltered lives, and the dead are hidden. The major adjustment to clinical medicine is to *see* death and dying.

I had never met the dead until Ellen, my cadaver. She smelled horrible, and she was no more humanoid than the cat I dissected in college. Familiarity with death began that first week in the dissecting room; often referred to as a dehumanizing process, the process of dissecting a corpse, living with the lingering odor in one's clothes and hair, being taught that we are reducible to an anatomy, is for many a jolting experience. This socialization to the world of medical objectification begins by recognizing that death is just another object of study, albeit a central one. Its scrutiny is inculcated into every aspect of medical education, and this then allows for an extrapolation from the dead to those with major or minor illness. The entire continuum of suffering was to be understood from the scientific perspective, where we were obviously dealing with persons, but in a most specific fashion: as objects of professional study.

For instance, our clinical language reinforced our distancing from the sufferer: We did not speak of the person, but of the case, the disease, the patient, the lesion, the abnormality, the anomaly, the surgery, the test result. We learned interview skills, how to glean the "relevant" clinical history. We sought *facts*, bits of objective information to be inserted into diagnostic equations. So in obtaining a "family history," we searched for genetic associated disease; our social histories documented whether our patient smoked, imbibed alcohol, worked. Travel history was also considered relevant, not so much to reflect the life-experience of our patient, but rather to ascertain risk factors for infection.

And of course the "best case" was the most perplexing, most difficult medical problem. The poor miserable soul who had suffered multiple trauma, five-system organ failure, or who required dialysis for drug overdose was only grist for our medical mill. It was very "challenging," and we students thoroughly reveled in the excitement, and importance, of our work. Medical school was difficult, but it was also enormous fun.

I graduated at the top of my class with an addendum to my name, M.D. My daughter, when young, referred to those initials as "my Daddy," denying, however mutedly, its other signification. Voicing her objection to sharing me with another world, she knew, as did the rest of the family, and as my father's wife and children knew before them, that M.D. also stood for "my destiny."

Joyce was in her early twenties and on a normal day would have been pretty. But she was not attractive today. Like a frightened animal, eyes wide, she was gasping for air. She had been breathing with difficulty for hours. She had suffered from asthma since childhood, and her medical chart was full, in many volumes, with the course of hospitalizations too numerous to count. She had come in again, unresponsive to home and then to emergency-room medications. I had been watching her closely for four hours and had reluctantly concluded that she would not respond to my armatarium. Despite my expertise in the biochemistry of asthma and acute allergy, I could not break the spasms. She simply could not breathe. I was frustrated. In truth, I was angry. I summoned the anesthesiologist on call to intubate her. We would use the course of last resort.

He was a resident, as I was. A bit dishevelled, probably from being on call all day and now beginning his all-night vigil. He quickly reviewed my notes and then went in to see Joyce. I assumed that the matter was in hand and I went on to other business. When I returned to the ward 45 minutes later, he was still in her room. Sitting by Joyce's bedside, he was just talking with her. I went in, and the gist of the monologue (for Joyce was not talking, but still gasping) was his reassuring her that she would be okay.

He stayed with her for three hours. Just talking. No more drugs, and of course no intubation. When he finally left around 2:00 a.m., she was breathing easily. As he passed me sitting at the nurses' station, he matter of factly noted that Joyce would require only some minor adjustments in her medications and should be ready for discharge the next day. He was right.

I flushed as I watched him walk down the hall. He had talked her out of the asthma attack. I recalled my anger at not being able to break the bronchoconstriction. I recoiled at the memory of my mother suffering irrational recalcitrance to therapies with her own asthma. I glanced at Joyce sleeping comfortably and I felt ashamed.

Some Definitions

- **ethics**—the discipline dealing with what is good and bad or right and wrong or with moral duty and obligation *(Webster's Third International Dictionary)*
- The "ought" is, in fact, one of the most common features of what "is," of what is happening. (John Caputo, *Against Ethics*)
- "How should one live?"—the generality of *one* already stakes a claim. (Bernard Williams, *Ethics and the Limits of Philosophy*)
- Moral responsibility . . . is the first reality of the self, a starting point rather than a product of society. . . . It has no "foundation"—no cause, no determining factor. . . . There is no self before the moral self, morality being the ultimate, nondetermined presence; indeed, an act of creation *ex nihilo*, if there ever was one. (Zygmunt Bauman, *Postmodern Ethics*)
- What we possess . . . are the fragments of a conceptual scheme, parts which now lack those contexts from which their significance derived. We possess indeed simulacra of morality, we continue to use many of the key expressions. But we have—very largely, if not entirely—lost our comprehension, both theoretical and practical, of morality. (Alasdair MacIntyre, *After Virtue*)

Before proceeding further, I wish to declare explicitly the strategies adopted for my argument. The first concerns the philosophical approach I have assumed in espousing a medical ethics. Contemporary ethics, as applied to various social questions, including those of bioethics generally and of medical ethics more narrowly, has witnessed a lively debate concerning the relation of "top-down" (deductive) versus "bottom-up" (inductive) approaches to its governing practice. On the first scheme, an overriding theory informs ethical principles, which then define the ethical rules that finally adjudicate particular cases. On the second approach, the process is reversed, with individual cases driving the process upward toward rules and principles, which finally materialize into an encompassing theory. Not surprisingly, a consensus appears to be emerging, according to which a combination of the approaches commands practice: Each level influences, but does not govern, the others. Norman Daniels calls this dialectical, bidirectional process "wide reflective equilibrium"—the slogan for a multifocal coherence of belief and practice.

To acknowledge both the plurality of approaches and the legitimacy of each is the triumph (and perhaps the failure) of late twentieth-century tolerance and eclecticism. Most practical medical ethicists adopt this pragmatic and effective approach, but moral philosophers generally build their theories from the most general considerations. I too will advocate a top-down approach. My argument does not even rest on principalism (the dominant school of medical ethics which has been characterized by Wayne Sumner and Joseph Boyle as having acquired "a virtually constitutional status in the bioethical realm"), but on a more overarching ethical theory. Principalism refers to the interplay of the key elements in American medical ethics, where these are taken to be autonomy, beneficence, nonmaleficence, and justice. One can hardly dispute these precepts, but I will argue for a more fundamental relational philosophy as preparatory to such supervening ethical principles and rules.

Second, I wish to place a self-reflexive ethics firmly in its social role. My thesis is that medicine's primary concern is ethical; science and technology must be placed in service to humane concerns. Medical ethics is not a subject among many to be taught in medical schools: it is *the* subject. And it is of paramount importance. Medical ethics is not simply jurisprudence applied for the protection of patients; it is a philosophical project whose foundations establish the relationships between health care providers and the ill. Medical ethics is not merely an apparatus placed in service of solving various technical issues; it is the very basis of how we approach and resolve the challenges offered by contemporary scientific achievements.

At the intersection of these two agendas—the primacy of my philosophical position and its social application—I wish to articulate a guiding *ethos* for contemporary medicine. The proposition I offer is on the one hand simple, a reassertion of a relational ethic as the foundation of medicine, yet on the other hand, the argument must be rigorously defended against competing philosophies of care. There are those who advocate the dominance of technological achievement, whose power and authority in dictating medical care has its own logic and priority. In that world of the technological imperative, relational ethics is subordinated to the science and technology that drive medical progress. Utility then becomes the guiding rationale, and the medical practitioner committed to that program is directed by the pragmatic results of his or her craft. On this view the patient should be satisfied with a highly sophisticated technology that has yielded increased longevity and quality of life. And when the discussion does drift to a concern for establishing a different framework for medical care, we hear dissension. There are those medical ethicists who maintain that medical care must be based on the same political ideals by which we fashion our liberal democracy. Others advocate a utilitarian approach. I will argue for a different, and I think more fundamental, basis for morality in the clinical setting.

The proposition I will advocate is hardly novel. In some other format the issue at hand might be referred to as the eclipse of compassion, and it is a problem that predates our modern era. Maimonides, writing in the twelfth century, cautioned that one should not engage in "speculation" (scientific inquiry) until one has "filled himself with the knowledge of what is forbidden and what is permitted." Simply, this Jewish philosopher reminded his medieval readers that moral standards and the cultivation of ethical behavior had priority over scientific practice. And many twentieth century commentators have repeated that assertion. For instance, Shimon Glick writes, "The foundation on which medicine must be based is compassion, that is where it all starts, and without this basis one cannot be a true physician." Not surprisingly, these testaments originate in a self-consciously religious orientation. Maimonides and Glick speak from the Jewish tradition; the virtue ethics of such prominent medical ethicists as Edmund Pellegrino, David Thomasma, and Albert Jonsen are the expres-

"Moral" pertains to the general domain of human relationships, and in this regard the Self is the moral vehicle that we employ to discuss how we ought to interact. Ethics becomes a metaphysical problem because the standards of such action are not derived from scientific knowledge or from any certainty that could be verified by Wittgensteinian standards of knowledge. We might well argue that it is immoral to murder, but that judgment is based on contentions fundamentally different in kind than those to which we can assign scientific objectivity. So to situate the Self in this moral cosmos is to acknowledge that we are discussing a construct that cannot fulfill the epistemological standards for scientific knowledge. Recall that from the Wittgensteinian perspective any discourse other than science is "nonsense"—which does not mean that we are indulging in silliness or stupidity, only that we must not mistake these discussions as entailing a standard of knowledge that can be attained. This is a simple admission, but it changes the exposition to a post-Wittgensteinian metaphysical formulation. So with this critical caveat, in this chapter I will turn unabashedly to metaphysics to articulate a response to this challenge of selfhood and its moral basis. Before doing so, let me briefly situate my argument.

Medical ethics comes in two kinds. One can only be called applied jurisprudence, which is the practical application of law and accepted practice. This is the variety that virtually any medical ethicist does, and it has specific areas of concern: (1) the physician-patient relationship (e.g., initiating and discontinuing the physician-patient relationship, confidentiality, informed consent, disclosure of information and truth-telling, assessing decision-making capacity, physician-patient sexual relations); (2) decisions near the end of life (surrogate decision-making, advance directives, withholding and withdrawing life-sustaining interventions, futile interventions, do-not-resuscitate orders, artificial nutrition and hydration, persistent vegetative state, brain death and determination of death, assisted suicide, active euthanasia, etc.); (3) the relationship of physician to society (e.g., access to health care and allocation of health resources, conflicts of interest, financial arrangements with HMOs, physician relationship to industry, advertising and marketing, capital punishment, impaired physicians); (4) ethical issues of physicians in training; (5) the role of ethics committees; and (6) research ethics (e.g., transplantation, protection of human subjects, genetic testing, unorthodox therapies). These are all highly practical and important areas of clinical medicine, and they increasingly help mold current practice.

But there is a second species of medical ethics, which is the attempt to define the philosophical basis of the medical encounter as a moral one. Medical ethics has quickly passed through three generations of development. The first was concerned with characterizing physicians' attitudes and reflections on ethical issues. This might be regarded as the coming-of-age or awareness phase. The second generation consisted of an analysis of ethical issues that gave rise to the technical discipline as described in the preceding paragraph. The third phase, the one I would call purely philosophical, is an attempt to situate medical ethics more broadly as a problem in general moral philosophy. (Several texts stand out as exemplars of this last genre, including *The Patient as Person* [1970] by Paul Ramsey, *Principles of Biomedical Ethics* [1979] by Tom Beauchamp and James Childress, *A Philosophical Basis of Medical Practice* [1981] by Edmund Pellegrino and David Thomasma, Robert Veatch's *A Theory of Medical Ethics* [1981] and H. Tristram Engelhardt, Jr.'s *The Foundations of Bioethics* [1996].) It is in this latter domain that the object of investigation broadens from patients' rights, clearly a worthwhile and significant matter, to the more fundamental ethical question of the *philosophical relation* of patient and health care provider. And in this context, the physician is no less a party to scrutiny than the object of his attention, the ill person. In other words, the ethical agent as well as the object of his ethical action must be examined. In this construction, the patient and his or her claims are no more prominent than the concern of defining the clinician as the moral agent and the relation between them. In simple terms, how the *physician* as a person—as a Self—deals with his or her patient becomes a crucial issue. Thus the problem of selfhood has been expanded from an issue for the patient alone to also encompass one for the physician.

Given that ethics is built upon the construction of a moral agent, and given the difficulty of defining the Self, how do we build a medical ethics? In attempting to answer this question, I admit to addressing only the second kind of medical ethics, for I am primarily concerned with the doctor-patient relationship. I believe it is to this encounter that we should devote our efforts in erecting a comprehensive philosophy of medicine that not only includes the aforementioned issues, but also situates the competing agendas of medical science and technology in their appropriate places. I maintain that discussions concerning our relation to science and technology are secondary to understanding the more fundamental moral concern of the Self-Other relationship. Our basis of knowing (our epistemology)— the science we rely upon to make informed and rational medical decisions—is not medicine, but only the tools of the discipline. Too often we confuse the technology and the science medicine employs as the discipline proper. The humanistic concerns are not mere appendages to the science of medicine in its various forms, but rather the very basis of medicine: medicine is grounded in the moral relationship of clinician and patient. The epistemology is subordinated to this relation.

The doctor was a priest in earlier times and remains so—albeit in a different guise—even now. Hospitals and clinics replete with diagnostic devices, surgical implements, drugs, etc.: These are the means by which care is given. Medical attention relies on this apparatus, but care is fundamentally ethical, that is, based on human relation. When we reorient our approach to medical ethics as a primarily moral venture, we will be in a better position to deal with the challenges posed by the awesome power of today's technology. In other words, we must firmly place medicine in its ethics, and the epistemology will follow in that service. My effort is then ultimately concerned with defining the Self in light of understanding the Self-Other relationship, from which an ethical foundation for medicine can be built.

Levinas

It was a cold day in March, and I was hurriedly walking down Newbury Street, the most fashionable street of Boston. There, sitting on the sidewalk was a black woman, huddled in a dark coat too big for her. As I passed, she plaintively cried, "Spare change?"

I glanced at her and didn't break stride for a few steps, then abruptly stopped and wheeled to face her.

"Carolyn! Carolyn, what the hell are you doing here?"

She looked up at me and an embarrassed half-smile cut across her face. A light in her eyes, the same intelligent light I had noted in the clinic on so many occasions, struck me as she wanly replied, "Hello, Dr. Tauber." She looked down.

"What's going on?"

Without lifting her head she matter-of-factly replied, "Well, I need money. The rent is due. I ran out."

I dug into my pocket and gave her a twenty-dollar bill. "Here, this is down payment for your next visit. Be sure to keep that appointment." I knew full well that there was at least a fifty percent chance she would not show up.

"Thanks, doc. I will."

And she did.

Fundamentally, to care for the patient is to place the Other in the focus of attention. Self-aggrandizement is subordinated, and the act of responsibility must dominate. The pledge often taken by graduating medical students, whether the Hippocratic Oath, the Maimonidean Physician's Prayer, or some other variant, is a pledge to care for others irrespective of any factor. A moral commitment made in the past projects into the future, guiding our behavior by assumed moral constraints. As Bernard Williams observed in *Ethics and the Limits of Philosophy,* "[O]bligation and duty look backwards, or at least sideways. The acts they require . . . lie in the future."

Perhaps obviously, I still believe and hope that medicine offers unique and ceaseless opportunities for exercising moral choices. Most health care providers are morally self-conscious, ever aware of their obligation. Perhaps sympathy or even empathy drives them, but I do not confuse these emotions with morality. And while I acknowledge the many masquerades of altruism and the various disguises we wear as health care professionals, there remains a deep moral commitment that situates our agency both in the clinic and at the bedside to guide our acts. As a physician, I cannot, just like the priest or judge in black, discard my white garb. This ancient costume defines me in a way that transfigures me to conform to an ethical mandate that I neither can escape nor forget, ministering to the ill as a fundamental act of response. By answering the other, I *am.* So my tack will be to go beyond autonomy as the basis of our ethical framework to plow the field of relational morality as a means toward our goal. It is the relational issue that will define our strategy.

The difficulty philosophy now has in contributing a general formulation of moral agency to the specific concerns of medical ethics has been clouded by a confusion of philosophy's own making. Perhaps for many overlapping and interwoven reasons, we find the problem of clearly presenting a philosophy of medical ethics compounded by a corresponding inability to articulate the parameters by which an ethical agent, the Self, may be formulated. In our preoccupation with identifying the Self, untethered and unstable, we have left in confusion not only the issue of how to construe moral agency: More generally, this philosophical unrest has left us bereft of a metaphysical grounding for our ethics. And it is this basic issue of selfhood that confuses us in our attempts to formulate a philosophy of medicine, and more particularly, to ground medical ethics firmly in a more comprehensive philosophy.

In large measure, the impediment to establishing a philosophy of medicine resides in the readily available philosophical "solution" to the issues of selfhood. Fundamentally, I believe that the contours of personhood comprise not an epistemological question, but a moral one. The deconstruction of the Self demands a moral response, and by shifting the discussion to this domain we enter into a different kind of analysis and a markedly altered conception of what it is to be an individual. As long as the Self remains in doubt, ill defined by the epistemological quandary of modern analytic thought, we will be thwarted in our efforts to find a firm foundation for medical philosophy, which I have already argued must be first and foremost an ethical philosophy. It seems to me that a crucial first step in articulating such a philosophy is to arrest the attack on the Self and to seek to salvage it as a vehicle for a moral philosophy.

So I now want to offer an intriguing solution to this problem, and I do so standing on the shoulders of a giant, Emmanuel Levinas, a French philosopher who died in 1995 at the age of ninety. Levinas argued with increasing authority that philosophy must address the individual's unavoidable responsibility for others. The Self is not only defined in relation to the Other, but the very nature of our being resides in that intersubjectivity. I offer an outline of his philosophy in the effort to construct an alternative to an autonomy-based ethic. I maintain that the grounding of medical ethics must account for both "selfness" and "relation," for on the foundation of a relational philosophy we will endeavor to build a comprehensive medical philosophy.

Levinas argues that the individual has an unavoidable responsibility for others. But his ethics takes on a much more global quality than a narrow construal of civic duty or moral attitude. His moral philosophy is a comprehensive view which plants epistemology (our knowledge of the world) and metaphysics (our basic conception of reality) in the ethical encounter. Thus the Self is not only defined in relation to the Other, but the Self becomes actualized in its very being in that intersubjectivity. For Levinas, *we are persons only in relation to our relationships with others.* This idea permeates his concept of being human. Levinas's philosophy is a radical response to a system of thought based solely on the autonomous moral agent. Since, as I have argued, medical ethics requires both "selfness" and "relation," Levinas's position is most intriguing and deserves careful scrutiny.

He begins by asking, What is the self and how is it constituted? In his view the Self discovers itself in alterity, in otherness. This is an intriguing idea, especially because there is a strong counterintuitive component to the argument. He does not begin with a self, but allows it to emerge or develop. In his perspective, the Self does not become a true self until it reflects upon its own selfhood. Like those nineteenth-century thinkers before him, Levinas is primarily concerned with our self-consciousness, the very act of contemplating our personal identities. But he takes this self-consciousness in a new direction by distinguishing two stages of thought, nonreflexive and reflexive.

Unless we consciously translate our thought process into linguistic terms, we can safely say that we think at a "preconscious" level as we act in the world. Perhaps an example will help illustrate the point: I hear a shriek and then a shout, "Dad, come quick!" Do I duly contemplate my surprise at my daughter's alarm, the linguistic content of her fear, or do I simply run with deliberate speed and attention to the kitchen where the shout originated? I arrive without "thinking" about my route, or any of the myriad details that compose the scene of my house and family in it. I see a fire on the stove. Do I consciously think of a my next action? Do I ponder, How do I put out this fire? Where is the extinguisher? No; I simply grab the fire extinguisher hung on the wall and hose down the flames. Later, I might reconstruct the entire episode, analyze its components and my reactions, and marvel at my adept handling of the emergency. In this sense, I behave *nonreflexively,* responding to my environment, acting with purpose and design, but with language never entering into my behavior. I did not articulate to myself "run down the stairs," or "move this leg then that leg," or "use the extinguisher on the wall above the sink," or any other command to engage in my spontaneous, noncontemplative actions.

But there is a second stage of thought, namely, self-awareness. Reading this book, thinking of questions and challenges to an elusive authorial agent who cannot respond directly and who controls the silent dialogue, is quintessentially reflexive. But I am not referring exclusively to rational thought, or even conscious thought dependent on language. I would include the global feelings we often call aesthetic, spiritual, or ethical—feelings that we find so difficult, if not impossible, to translate into linguistic terms. When discussing or expressing these states, we are very aware that translation must occur, and like all translation it is both incomplete and distorted in respect to the original. Translation cannot be identical to what it translates. So language *per se* is not the *sine qua non* of reflexive thought; self-awareness is.

Thus we must distinguish a consciousness that does not "think" but "lives" nonreflexively. This distinction is aptly illustrated by the difference between getting on a bicycle and riding down the street, and teaching someone how to first master the same procedure. In the first instance, we just *do* it; in the second, we have to break down the act into its various components, explaining the tricky nature of starting off, attaining velocity, keeping balance, braking, and the various other nuances of what we skilled peddlers take for granted. We use language to describe how it feels to compensate our balance, but ultimately we know that our student will simply have to intuit the right action with our rather ponderous and inarticulate advice.

Thought then begins with reflection on primordial consciousness, and in this thought the outside world then becomes articulated: it is non-Self. Thought presents to itself what is extrinsic to it, and perception and appropriation of our perceived world is defined by this self-consciousness. To be human, for Levinas, is to have the ability to separate ourselves from the world, to self-reflect on our very consciousness. This act of contemplating our "Self," that which distinguishes us as perceiving and feeling beings, is the basis of our humanity. The "Other" then becomes the crucial catalyst of the Self. Alterity is established only in the nonreciprocity of relation, in the "foreignness" of the Other. In the radical separation *and* relation with the Other, produced simultaneously, the subject becomes a "host," or in the vocabulary we have been using, a true *Self*. This is a key step in erecting Levinas's ethical framework: the Self must and can only exist in response to the Other.

The Self lives in a continuously contextual perspective. We are all in fact together in the world. It is through others' responses that I get a sense of the quality of my own being; moreover, in carrying out my own projects, I inevitably impinge on the world of others. As intentional activity, consciousness makes itself *be* by its choice of action in the world. So before free will and self-responsibility, we must recognize the world of others and our relation to it. This self-awareness is then the origin of epistemology for Levinas. To *know* the world is to be self-conscious of our knowing; and to be so aware, we must acknowledge our separate natures, Self and Other.

For Levinas, *relation*, or the intersubjective in the social domain, thus actualizes the self. The will of Nietzsche no longer suffices to define the Self. In a sense, the vital Self—the unconscious, nonreflexive Self, the Nietzschean will—is only a prelude to the Self that recognizes itself through the Other. According to this scheme, one's ethical relation to the Other is ultimately prior even to his relation to himself or to the totality of things that we call the world. Truly to encounter another as a stranger, unknown and irreducible to ourself, forces us to place everything that *we* are into question. This encounter is the essential challenge of selfhood. As we recognize the Other, the non-Self, we discover ourselves.

That discovery has no *required* ethical structure. Why not just murder the Other? All too often that, of course, occurs. Our own century has witnessed the most horrendous mass murders in history—the Armenian genocide, the Soviet communization, the Jewish Holocaust, the Chinese cultural revolution, the Cambodian atrocity, the Rwandan butchery—on and on. Levinas would be hard pressed to say that the status of otherness *per se* confers any moral standing, considering the horrific experience of murder in our own time, where being an "other" seems to confer a ticket to oblivion.

Even in more civil contexts, we are struck by the latitude of our moral codes. Whatever realm of society we examine, these same questions arise. For instance, in business it is commonplace to take advantage where one can. We admire the shrewd businessman who buys low and sells high. That is the mark of robust capitalism, but the line between good business practice and exploitation is often blurred, and we have consumer protection agencies to protect the innocent or ignorant, too often unaware of his victimization. But we need not look far for other examples. How often do we make ethnic jokes, or make fun of some minority group? Hiding income at tax time seems to be a national sport. And what about "trivial" infractions like cutting in the traffic line, forgetting to return that borrowed book—or keeping the patient waiting just to enjoy a second cup of coffee, or postponing a response to the night bell from that fussy man in room 11?

Levinas is neither naive nor quixotic. He maintains that ethical behavior must arise from two sources, one metaphysical (and I postpone discussion of that until later), and the other social. Moral behavior results from recognizing that the Self is essentially engaged in the world and is responsible for what both itself and the world become. Ethical responsibility to others rests on the recognition that in acting in the world, one inevitably changes it for others as well as for oneself. So the intersubjective encounter both affords self-definition—in itself an ethical act—and demands response in a world now consisting of a contextualized self.

Psychologically, the goal is to secure one's own being. The person who cherishes the illusion of being only a subject precludes the possibility of interrelation or growth from contact with others, for in such encounters, we must recognize that we become objects too. It is on this incessant dialectical engagement of *self* and *other*, where each is defined by the other, that we must focus our own project. We are all both subjects and objects.

In a caring world, to which we all presumably aspire (a huge assumption to be sure), the exchange must become the mutual pledge and invitation to respect each other's subjectivity, and our respective identities. Levinas has pointed out how such a project is to be approached—alterity (otherness) begets personhood through responsibility. This is the crucial twist to the notion of encounter: The Self is defined not simply by the Other, but by its *responsibility* for the Other.

This brings us back to our earlier concerns about the living subject, what we have called the Self. Living nonreflexively in the world, we are unaware of our individuality. Only by contemplating our identity do we become aware of our distinctness from and our place within the world. The provocation of Levinas's thought rests on the following delicate point: the Self is not turned in upon itself (that is, forced to consider the separateness of its being) until confronted by the Other. And then a remarkable recognition occurs, as we perceive the extraordinary richness and potential of each relationship. The very uniqueness of each encounter makes its impression on us, and as we are contextualized and turned out of ourselves into relation, we see our own reflection in the Other. To *see* another then becomes an ethical act. Why its arrow is toward the good rather than evil is a metaphysical concern which I will leave for the last chapter, but suffice it here to note that in medicine the moral structure is given. *Empathetic care is prescribed in the role of the health care provider, and thus the ethical vector is established.* We need not worry about seeking the basis for the ethical relation of recognizing the Other: in the clinical setting it is there from the first encounter. We just need to be reminded of that existential fact.

5

Toward a New Medical Ethic

He was screaming. He had been screaming for three days. Sometimes he would only moan, but usually he was yelling. The tumors had infiltrated his skull. The radiotherapists could not give him any more treatment, and anesthesia could not give a sectional block. We were left with narcotics alone, and the drugs were not sufficient. Everyone was complaining, but there was nothing to be done.

It was midnight, and Mrs. Murphy, the head nurse, took me aside. "Are you the intern responsible for Mr. Levenger?"

"Yes."

"What are you going to do about him?"

"I don't know what to do. The drug orders are written. Morphine drip to keep comfortable."

"That's all?"

"What else can we do?"

Mrs. Murphy turned on her heel and went to the narcotics cabinet. She unlocked it with the keys dangling at her side. Filling a syringe, she locked the door again and walked down the hall to Mr. Levenger's room. The door had been closed, and upon opening it, the muffled noise suddenly become louder and clearer. The door then closed again. Five minutes later Mrs. Murphy emerged and strode back to the ward desk.

"Mary, call the morgue, housekeeping, and admissions. You," pointing to me, "better go pronounce Mr. Levenger and call the family." She then went into the nurses' lounge, sat down and lit a cigarette. She scribbled her notes in the chart, and then put her head down in her arms. When I went to retrieve the chart to write my own death note, I first read hers.

"Patient found apneic and pulseless at 12:12 A.M. Code not called per physician orders. Doctor notified."
I then wrote my note.

I have found that my role as philosophical or historical commentator usually elicits comments of "interesting" or "fascinating" or some such noncommittal nod to my perspective. Some are less charitable. The chairwoman of our medical school curriculum committee, Dr. Q., recently said to me, "Our students are not interested in philosophy, and it only confuses them." I am becoming increasingly dissatisfied with dismissal. Philosophy should be taken seriously, and in my frustration I have often fantasized of handing out tee-shirts to our entering medical students: In bright colors on the front I would have emblazoned the slogan, "Medicine *must* become philosophical," with an imprint of Locke or Hume or Kant or Nietzsche on the back. A gesture, no doubt, and a rather feeble one, no more persuasive than the bumper sticker "I brake for animals," nor more informative than "This car climbed Mt. Washington." Yeah, so what. But my tee-shirt is just the launching pad for my vision, and then I let my imagination fly. Let's revise the curriculum! The first thing to do is fire Dr. Q. and her entire committee! A wonderful thought. Then as my reverie goes forward, I come up against certain uncomfortable realities, the first of which is that I would also have to replace the Associate Dean of Admissions.

Perhaps Dr. Q is right; our medical students are not philosophical. After all, they have been selected to perform in a certain way. So, we must redefine our admissions requirements. But why stop there? We need curricular reform in college. If we want candidates who have exhibited the intellectual and humanistic qualities of a Pope John XXIII or Martin Luther King, Jr., then students must be encouraged to excel in community service, and to take college courses to stimulate their philosophical development. Ah, the task grows, as I imagine a dramatic reinforcement of moral and intellectual orientation sharply distinct from that dominating our medical centers today. I soon become quite discouraged by my own grandiose dreams. But there are immediate sensitivities that might be encouraged. To these I now turn.

I think that some perspective on the limits of our knowledge and an examination of medicine's logic and decision making are crucial lessons to be learned by all physicians. But I am not referring narrowly to instruction or some curricular reform here. More pointedly, I am advocating a self-conscious metaphysical examination. Medicine is already sufficiently scientific and technical; what it lacks is the perspective of directly dealing with its broader humanistic concerns. What I mean is that health practitioners must be committed to a continuous self-assessment of their role as care-givers. This is a moral activity, and as such, it is deeply metaphysical.

It is commonplace to speak of medicine as an ethical venture, whose moral responsibilities of caring for the ill are complicated by a science that continuously amazes us with its power to cure and its sophistication to analyze, leading us to complex ethical decisions. When do we stop life support systems? What are the legal rights of surrogate mothers? Should we genetically modify our reproductive germ cells to prevent genetic disease? How do we regulate organ donations? As important as such questions might be, I am not concerned here with the particulars of medical ethics. In a sense, I even admit to not being so interested in medical ethics as usually understood. I am, however, deeply interested in medicine becoming more self-consciously moral.

It is no surprise that medical ethics is a growing field that has come to dominate discussions of medicine's moral concerns. After all, with the new challenges brought on by our technical advances and the potential applications of molecular biology, we are continually faced with radically new ethical challenges. In this crucible of change, we have witnessed the birth of medical ethics as a subspecialty, a discipline with its own expertise and responsibilities. The questions medical ethicists ponder, and for the most part effectively address, certainly require answers. We need people to deal with these issues, and I would not in any way denigrate them or their efforts. Certainly, we profit from their teaching. But in another sense, I regard medical ethicists as part of medicine's larger crisis, and not necessarily its solution as currently constituted. The problem I address may be seen quite clearly in the recognition that "medical ethics" has become a specialty of experts.

In the professionalization of the discipline we witness the growth of a highly specialized language and system of rewards developed for its practitioners as in any other self-interested academic field. Perhaps one should not be surprised, but when I read recently about the Third Inter-Collegiate Ethics Bowl I must admit to some incredulity. At the 1997 annual meeting of the Association for Practical and Professional Ethics, fourteen teams representing various colleges and universities were posed questions relating widely to professional ethics and social and political morality. The University of Montana apparently "won." How does one *win* a contest in ethics? What could be the standard canon of referral, the recently published *Encyclopedia of Applied Ethics*? Should we have specialty bowls for medical ethics alone? Probably, and then we will move from the playful to the serious: Eventually, no doubt, there will be specialty boards in medical ethics, complete with right and wrong type exams. At last we will then have a mechanism of certifying Plato's Philosopher Kings. I must demur.

All health care providers must become ethicists. I as a doctor feel that each physician must self-consciously recognize the moral obligations—and, indeed, opportunities—of caring for the ill. Ethics in medicine has always been assumed. Now it has become explicit as a "problem," but not simply in the narrow way that experts in medical ethics worry about. We must recognize in training young health care workers that merely knowing some medical ethical statute such as informed consent is not enough to be able to discuss this concept effectively with a patient. Nor does mere education in medical ethics more broadly guarantee humane care to best serve medical or moral ends. My solution, to the extent that I am brazen enough to formulate one, is that medicine must not "attach" ethics to its practice or science, but must recognize that ethics dominates all its endeavors. Medicine is fundamentally ethical and should be recognized as such. Unfortunately, medical ethicists too often teach another lesson altogether. For instance, Howard Brody writes in *Ethical Decisions in Medicine*, that "medical ethics is not a branch of medicine, but a branch of ethics." He thus plainly commits us to continued segregation of ethics as an applied discipline and thereby perpetuates the artifical separation of clinical medicine from its ethics. *Ethics peripheral to medicine is our quandary, and the solution is the total integration of clinical practice with its attendant moral philosophy.*

I am skeptical about the prospects for teaching moral sensitivity, which includes not only knowledge of medical ethics *per se*, but also a compassionate attitude toward the suffering. One deliberate attempt at this might be an effort to select carefully those individuals with the requisite sensitivity and maturity to be empathetic and to endeavor to train them to maximize these faculties. Much might be accomplished by reinforcing character traits that are otherwise stifled. Can we prioritize the *humane* care of the ill, and teach this in the classroom, in the clinic, and at the bedside? I am not sanguine about the possibilities. There are no real solutions of this kind, because we are swimming against a mighty social tide. Before me, other physicians (like Seymour Glick writing in the 1981 *New England Journal of Medicine*) and philosophers (like David Roochnik writing in his 1987 *Philosophy in Context*) have commented that professionals largely reflect the society that trained them and in which they absorbed their values. Exhibiting a certain cultural persona, a beginning medical or nursing student has moral attitudes that are already well established, and these of course have been gleaned from various sources—family, school, religious community, and perhaps most pervasive, culture at large. Ethics of the kind I am advocating cannot be taught, enforced, or imposed upon adults, though we can reinforce those ethical inclinations that might be cultivated to blossom in full array. But in the end, we must hope for and rely on the self-selecting demands of medicine's moral calling beyond such nurturing. And as gatekeepers, we must choose those who recognize the crisis in which we are living as a deeply moral challenge. Embedded in our own time, I cannot clearly see how the social drama that was described earlier may play out on this terrain. Perhaps the very forces that are driving medicine ostensibly in one direction will be effectively galvanized by those committed to another ideal. I fervently hope so, and I have tried in this essay to state those choices clearly.

Perhaps the question of situating ethics in medicine is not so new. In a sense, the ingredients for this development have always been with us. Medicine is lodged firmly between two domains: the moral (what is right) and the epistemological (how we know what we think we know). That is to say, the complex enterprise that we call medicine is made up of two kinds of activities, two obviously connected but different modes of thought and action. Medicine claims its epistemological legitimacy in science, and it is as a science that modern clinical care is usually measured. The rise of scientific medicine in the nineteenth century and its fulfillment in the twentieth represent a major triumph of scientific ideals and the promise of its methods. Modern medicine is a major, if not *the* chief, beneficiary of science.

Although science has dominated most domains of medicine, there is a more ancient concern of medicine, and that is the care of the patient. This is what I refer to as the moral dimension, and it is here that the deepest commitment of medicine resides. As a moral activity, medicine *employs* science for its purposes. But make no mistake of the order of action: the moral precedes the epistemological. Failure to understand this, and more fundamentally failure to recognize the dominance of the ethical over the epistemological, is the root of our current confusion. But this is not to say that there is an inherent contradiction between being scientific and being compassionate. Technology is, and should be, placed in the service of human need. It is absurd to argue about "technology gone rampant." It is *we* who decide on the use of machines and drugs, and it is our collective voice that determines how we will use the products of scientific inquiry. As C. S. Lewis wrote in *The Abolition of Man* (1947), "What we call man's power over nature turns out to be a power experienced by some men over other men, with nature as its instrument." My point (and Lewis's) is simply that we must deliberately decide on the character of that use. Technology is itself neither moral nor immoral, only people are.

We might better understand this central matter by specifically addressing the relation of ethics to medicine as a science, as an epistemology. Medicine is of course constructed in some way from both domains; but more to the point, the sum of these domains cannot neatly categorize such a complex activity as medicine. The relationship between ethics and epistemology is not fixed, and each endeavor is in a sense framed by the other; but I am advocating a philosophy that is based not on medicine's epistemology, but instead on its ethics. In short, I enjoin us all to ponder the possibility of ethics as *the* priority for a philosophy of medicine.

To restate the overarching question, the essential philosophical challenge in modern medicine is to resolve how medicine goes beyond science and technology to reaffirm its humane concerns. Obviously doctors are committed to truth and to establishing rational therapies, but the problem is how to place our science in its proper role. The origin of our modern predicament may be traced to the seventeenth century, as the study of the human body demanded the objectification of ourselves, as objects of scientific inquiry. As discussed in chapter 1, this project was conceptually completed in the course of the nineteenth century, when medicine struggled effectively to claim scientific objectivity. This was the program enunciated by the Parisian physicians who sought to correlate anatomic pathology with clinical disease, and later by the German physiologists, who proudly proclaimed their reductionist research agenda to purge physiology and medicine of any vestiges of vitalism. Life processes were to be reduced to their most elemental physics and chemistry. The gains are self-evident, and the power of modern biochemistry and molecular biology are the just desserts of this approach.

But there is another compelling issue to address: Illness is dehumanizing. The Self becomes damaged, and the task is to restore the patient's full sense of identity. The medical scientist might be satisfied with "patient-as-disease," but the caring physician is guided by her recognition of the suffering person *in toto*. Analysis of the medical encounter must be based on viewing the patient not as a "case," a diseased entity, but as an experiencing, in fact suffering, individual. Being ill alters our very selfhood, changing our fundamental relationship to our own bodies. The ill lose freedom through impairment. The patient's dependence upon others for recovery, and hence his or her loss of freedom, results in increased vulnerability and consequently weakened self-image. We must adopt a medical ethics that recognizes as a first principle the humanity of the ill.

Now, those with even a passing acquaintance with discussions addressing these issues might rightly note that this appraisal is hardly novel. But the point I wish to make is not that we have failed to recognize the problem of dehumanization and of how to construct an ethics to correct it, but rather *why* we are having so much difficulty effectively addressing this moral crisis. If we essentially agree that a technocratic medicine is dehumanizing at precisely the point in a patient's life when he or she most needs humane care, then why haven't we "fixed" the problem? Because, I think, we need first to properly identify the issues.

We make a damaging category mistake when we fail to distinguish medicine from its supporting sciences, which are a critical component of medicine's mission but hardly its sole means. When we confuse the enormous growth in scientific medicine with medicine proper, we approach hubris, on the one hand, claiming to know that illness *is* simply physico-chemical disruption, and on the other, we short-change medicine's caring mission. In the scientific achievements of applied biology and chemistry, medicine's fundamental ethos was to a large extent usurped by another ideal, the reduction of disease to the gene or its substituted basic element. The patient became a scientific object, and the ethical relation of the healer to the individual in need was fundamentally altered.

"I saw a great case today."

"Yeah."

"This guy comes in with nondescript fatigue. I checked him out. He had these really faint lines under his nails."

"Yeah."

"Well, yeah. He had splinter hemorrhages! And he had a murmur! The son-of-a-bitch has endocarditis!"

"Wow! What did Dr. Meier think?"

"You know. He went into orbit. We're getting a whole bunch of tests and Infectious Diseases will see him this afternoon. I'm so psyched."

The patient is all too easily reduced to an object of interest, albeit to honest and good purpose. But ultimately, we should seek a clinical science that treats *persons,* not diseases. To counter what might be called "radical objectification," we must consciously instate ethics as a crucial constituent of medical theory and practice. No longer an appendage or subject among others, ethics must take center stage to direct its supporting cast of medical sciences. In short, our priority must be to focus upon medicine's original moral mandate.

How do we do this? Not by reaffirming the ethical principles that have dominated discussion in recent years. We have been so preoccupied with establishing those parameters by which patient autonomy will be respected, through what may broadly be referred to as judicial constraints or guidelines, that a thorough examination of the philosophical basis of the physician's ethical relation to the patient pleads for attention. As my colleague David Roochnik observed to me, "We need ethics . . . but all we have is autonomy, and that's not enough." Doctors, in identifying themselves so thoroughly as scientists or as technocrats, have lost their fundamental ethical moorings. Too many are so estranged from their patients that they must self-consciously seek guidance, directives, orders, and shared responsibilities to practice ethically. Granted, there are complex cases where judicial direction is essential, but too often the reliance on others for ethical guidance reflects a loss of the basic intuition of care.

The Commonwealth demands that we take risk management courses in which lawyers lecture us. The medical community embraces these so-called remedies as part of a defensive reaction to an outraged and bitter public seeking remunerative revenge for medical malpractice (certainly justifiedly) but, more deeply, expressing dissatisfaction with the very character of medical practice. When I embarked on my medical career twenty-five years ago, malpractice suits were rare. Why? Not because physicians were any more technically competent or diligent. The basic reason was that patients trusted and respected their doctors, and if things went badly it was typically understood, based on an implicit and reasonable trust, that the doctor had done his or her best and that sometimes bad things happen. Medicine has certainly been caught in our contemporary society's preoccupation with liability and litigation, but the physician might have remained immune. Something profoundly disruptive broke the public's trust. I look for the offending germ in the confusion over medicine's mission.

The signs are obvious to all of us. Physicians are instructed in medical jurisprudence, not ethics. Jurisprudence is situated in an intrinsically adversarial context: litigation and the courts. Our medical students and residents are given survey lectures to learn medical ethics—actually medical law. Medical ethics has become one subject among many taught in medical schools and a tag or an appendage to the health care industry. Like any industry in our society, this too needs careful governance to protect its consumers. Because patients do not trust their physicians as they did a generation ago, physicians have largely lost their professional autonomy. Doctors (and for that matter, nurses and other health care providers) must be warned of their potential liabilities, the administrative measures which must be taken to protect themselves (yes, protect!), and the legal limits on the exposure of their supporting institutions must be explained. I have been tortured by all-day seminars devoted to these matters, and I attended not because I thought the activity was intrinsically worthwhile, nor that such a didactic lesson was efficient, nor because I was challenged or fearful of the challenges to which I must respond, but rather because I was forced to, as a requirement of being a member of my hospital group. I chafed at these "solutions," which were only manifestations of the problem. Beyond the social and economic repercussions of the changes evident in the evolution of modern medicine, we are witness to a markedly altered ethical relationship between patient and healer. To attend these classes was only to be reminded in vivid detail the dimensions of our moral morass.

In many respects, it is right that the physician-as-god should fade from our collective memory, but with what model has it been replaced? Please note: the physician's power, for all of its dangerous implications, still demanded the physician's responsibility. If the physician is now to share responsibility with other members of the health provider complex, what remains as the basis of his moral commitments and how is it to be defined? Traditionally, physicians were regarded as having fiduciary responsibility for their patients. The law defines a fiduciary as a person entrusted with power or property to be used for the benefit of another and legally held to the highest standard of conduct. But as Marc Rodwin notes, although doctors perform fiduciary-like roles and hold themselves out as fiduciaries in their ethical codes, today the law regards such a fiduciary function only in restricted situations. "Fiduciary" is now in fact a metaphor and no longer has much application to the doctor-patient relationship, which for me, at least, is a startling revelation. While the doctor-patient relationship presupposes entrusting physicians to act on their client's behalf, fiduciary principles have only been applied for very limited purposes: physicians cannot abandon their patients, they must keep clinical information confidential, and they must disclose to patients any financial interest in clinical research. As Rodwin explains, the ambiguity arises because

there is no equivalent for physicians of the conflict-of-interest prohibitions that exist for most fiduciaries. Malpractice law could hold physicians liable for departing from broad fiduciary standards, if such standards existed; yet they do not. Malpractice law—which holds physicians responsible for their negligence— only adumbrates fiduciary standards. It focuses on physicians' technical competence . . . [and] traditional fiduciary responsibilities. But only a small part. Generally malpractice law ignores traditional fiduciary concerns. ("Strains in the Fiduciary Metaphor")

I find it telling that a patient's legal recourse is almost always channeled through charges of negligence, not through fiduciary responsibility, as this reveals that the law recognizes the weakness of moral responsibility as a guiding ethos for the doctor-patient relationship. Simply put, doctors generally are not held accountable, other than as technicians who must perform up to the community standard. Undoubtedly this is a critical basis for practice, but it is woefully inadequate as a moral code. The legal model of malpractice, self-protective and adversarial, is obvious evidence of failure.

With the growing institutionalization of medicine, physicians will have increasingly divided loyalties as they act as gatekeepers, rationing medical resources for the benefit of providers, insurers, the government, or society at large. Their tasks include limiting specialty referrals, certifying eligibility for disability income or insurance benefits, and admitting patients to the hospital or intensive care units based on clinical criteria as well as other than strict medical need. Quality reviewers are establishing protocols to set the parameters of medical attention; third-party payers establish policies on what services are provided, the rates of reimbursement, and the standards of care. What doctors do clinically has become a complex calculus of weighing benefits for the individual patient against the aims and performance of amorphous managed care organizations. As Rodwin observes, and as I lament, patients are but "one of the many parties that have a claim on physicians' loyalty, but not one that overrides the claims of other parties." The very structure of what may fairly be called the medical-industrial complex is so determined by its economic operations that physicians are in fact beholden to forces that intervene between himself or herself and the patient.

This highly complex legal issue has convoluted social and economic aspects, but ultimately it only can reflect—and be subordinated to—the deeper ethical issue with which we are preoccupied. The limited applicability of the physician's fiduciary function reflects the deep quandary into which we have fallen. The restrictions of accountability illustrate two cardinal features of our medical system: (1) the reliance on legal autonomy—and self-responsibility—of the patient, and (2) the divided loyalty of physician responsibility. The result is the same despite the different origins of the social forces: Positivist science objectifies disease to the extent of reducing patients to "cases" and treating them as objects of research; HMOs sacrifice humane, totalyzing care for efficiency and investment return. Science and technology have usurped the traditional and sustaining ethos of medicine, and our economic health-care delivery system has reinforced the patient's "objectification." Each reduces the patient to an object—in one case, a scientific curiosity, in the other, an entity to be marketed to and then efficiently processed. In both contexts, autonomy—assuming somewhat different guises—serves the respective agenda by forfeiting a more comprehensive ethic.

I maintain that medicine must lay claim to its prior agenda and radically reorient itself to its defining moral mandate—the *interaction* of physician and patient, the basis of the healing art in all cultures. Science and technology, preoccupied with different concerns, may indeed come into play, but they must be subordinated to medicine's own program of placing the relation of patient and healer at the center of its praxis. Economic restraints must be dealt with, but perhaps our current system has become too restrictive and now requires a radical reassessment to the end of giving physicians more authority and latitude than currently allowed. I cannot address the particulars of either case and must be content with the philosophical project, but I trust that a self-conscious philosophical appreciation of the issues will help clarify our perplexity and stratify some practical solutions. To this moral project we now turn.

Much has been written about how a humanistic medicine views the patient in his or her entirety, how the sufferer is poorly served in a depersonalizing environment. Accounts are legion of the distress endured by patients in the contemporary clinic and hospital. I see it myself daily. We are, however, baffled as to what to do. When I speak to colleagues, peers, and younger doctors-in-training, the usual reply is that we are subject to market forces beyond our control, that the effort both to survive professionally and to serve our patients as best we can requires juggling skills with great dexterity and finesse. Physicians are disheartened, for there is general discouragement that we can effect change. Largely disenfranchised, our ability to alter the system is increasingly thwarted. As employees, we have little to say any longer in key management decisons. Coupled with the scientific ethos I have described, today's physician, despite what I believe is a generally held sincere wish "to do good," is poorly situated to practice medicine humanistically. So, despite all the discussion about humanizing medicine, there are precious few prescriptions for its implementation. Frustration is moving quickly toward despondency. Some of my colleagues have joined the "enemy" and gone into administration; others have retired early; a few, like me, have become commentators; but most, the vast majority, stay put, dispirited if not angry that the promise of medicine is not being realized in a country of such wealth and prosperity.

Despite the deeply embedded influences that have contributed to our lapse of moral fervor, I believe that the patient may again become the true and undivided object of responsibility. No one argues against the physician's being scientifically and economically responsible, but after ensuring those functions, why not insist that there is an even more fundamental demand: he or she must act as a moral agent. Now, an important caveat: I am not advocating a return to paternalism. The physician's expertise grants no moral or political superiority. But at the same time, there is no parity between the roles of the healer and the ill. It is the doctor's moral responsibility to exercise his or her superior knowledge in the effort to restore patient autonomy; this is quite different from saying that the doctor has free rein in the relationship. So to argue for a "relational philosophy" does not mean that such a relation is symmetrical. Our fear of losing our autonomy makes us alert to any infringement, but to be ill is already to admit our selfhood has been compromised. The patient, then, enters into a relation with the healer not as an equal—but does so in the hope of regaining his or her autonomy and equality.

From this perspective we can now ask, Where might the notion of an ethical medicine situate itself within the ethos of a reductionist science and a cost-effective business environment? How will a scientifically dominated medicine comprehensively and effectively incorporate the ethical position as fundamental to practice?

If one posits that the relation between doctor and patient has been critically wounded, how are we to understand whether, and on what basis, this relationship may be reasserted as foundational? In short, how might such a formulation serve as the grounding for a philosophy of medicine? I maintain that if we were to accept the centrality of a relational moral philosophy within medicine, we would be dealing with a potentially radical and far-reaching proposal. For to argue that medicine has an ethical meta-physics is first to claim that the very basis of medicine is to find and assert its own philosophy in the context, not of science or competing economic demands, but in the care of the patient. As Norman Levinsky has written, the patient must again be recognized as the physician's master.

The Call of the Other

From Locke to Levinas! How might we begin to fill in a philosophy of medicine along such a taut manifold? I believe it is precisely upon this tension that such a philosophy must be erected. The conflict in fact begins at their common point—the self. Each seeks to identify the basis of the unity of the self, and to dispel those attempts that would disallow such a being. This is a crucial principle for them to hold in common, especially now when the very legitimacy of selfhood has become highly problematic. The implications are profound for *any* ethics, for a responsible agent must be a *self*, an integrity of being, to participate in any ethical dialogue.

We must find a synthesis for the ethical enterprise on a dipole that encompasses two distinct (albeit overlapping) positions. At the first pole resides the autonomous agent. This is the commonly held view of selfhood, woven from a densely textured matrix dealing with questions of individual autonomy and self-reliance, which have served as the foundation of many bioethical philosophies. The contrasting pole upholds the relational aspect of self, the "otherness" of responsibility. The most obvious—and most important—point to be made here is that in medicine, the "problem"—and I put the word in scare quotes—of the Other vanishes. Taking Levinas's position, we become selves in a mutual encounter *with* the Other. On this humane view, unlimited autonomy is a mark of irresponsibility. In some contexts the Other is the despised, the debased, the demeaned. The foreignness of the Other then is seen as pejorative, a reflexion of the practical limits of Levinas's ethics. But the Other may also exist as an attribute, as an engaging opportunity, as a wonder. Medicine begins with the Other's character already resolved. By dictate, by fiat, by assumption, the Other *qua* patient is ultimately defined by the ethical responsibility accepted and embraced by the healer. Physicians and nurses are in principle committed to the care of the patient, and in this fundamental sense, the health care provider is defined by this responsibility. Thus Levinas's critics who decry his inability to effectively deal with the possibility of the Other as evil, at least in the domain of medicine, find no firm footing. The Other in the medical scenerio is given as the object of care. His status as good or evil is in principle moot.

Of the many World War II stories my father often told us, the morality play he struggled with most was the case of the Hungarian official brought to him before the Budapest Jews were submitted to the terrors of deportation and concentration camps. The man required emergency surgery, and my father performed the operation without complication, saving the gentile's life. Even knowing the politics of his patient and his likely role in tormenting Jews, my father had no compunction about performing at the peak of his professional competence.

Soon after, the patient supervised the rounding up of many of my father's compatriots and personally murdered several of them. He led a band of roving Hungarian fascists, who took hapless Jews still awaiting trains bound for death camps and summarily dispatched them into the Danube River with a bullet to the head. Tormented by the irony of his position, my father explained his lack of choice . . . the moral predicament allowed no latitude. His anguish was obvious; his purported certainty was never convincing. I only listened.

Levinas's ethical portrait offers a focus of concern that has shifted from the patient alone, that is, the autonomous subject, to the patient's relation to the doctor. And in this shift we are offered a new perspective, where medical ethics realigns the manner in which we might construct a philosophy of medicine. Physicians and nurses wear white, which in this case is an interesting contrast to the priesthood—opposite and yet the same. Doctors as healing priests, dressed in white, have heard the summons to become healers. Assuming this calling, this responsibility, it forms their existential character. They in fact *are* defined by their Other—the patient. Fundamentally, for the healer there is no choice—his or her calling is this ethical self-definition.

I learned this lesson at an early age under special circumstances. My father was my doctor. His father had died in World War I, when mine was only

18 months old. My grandfather saw him only once, briefly in a train station on his way to the Russian front. Whether he was killed or captured and sent to Siberia, no one knew for sure. My father made certain that I always knew where—and who—he was.

He always teased me that I received his medical attention for free. I never quite understood the joke. He gave me penicillin injections, and cleaned my wounds from war games and "battles" on the street. At age five when I required a tonsillectomy, I insisted he perform the surgery; only years later did he confess that another surgeon did the operation. When I fractured my wrist, he set the bones, and when I had hepatitis he supervised my care. I never doubted his expertise, trusting him completely. It is most natural for me to think of medicine as essentially relational; after all, my doctor was my father. But it seems to me that this primary relation can be, in fact is, universalized in medicine.

The cover illustration chosen for this book is Sir Luke Fildes' The Doctor. *This Victorian pastoral drama shows a country doctor sitting contemplatively at the bedside of a sick child, whose parents look on in dismay and fear. Portraying the medical reality of that period just before the explosion of scientific medicine, Fildes' evocation of the empathetic doctor, helpless in the face of nature's ravage and yet steadfastly committed to remaining with his young patient, both reflected the sentimentality of that era and also stated clearly the ethical relationship of the physician to his charge. Enormously popular, the painting was copied as a steel engraving in 1893 by Thomas Agnew and Sons, and several years ago I purchased the last copy of that original run from the London publishing house. It hangs on my study wall today. I have had a long, personal relationship with the picture. A pharmaceutical house had distributed color versions for doctors' offices, and my father had a copy that I loved to study. Knowing my attachment to this lithograph hanging in his waiting room, he gave me a small three-dimensional porcelain facsimile of the scene—also supplied by the drug company. It sat on my nightstand for years, and I often contemplated its pathos. Today, the painting still occupies a prominent place at the Tate Gallery in London, and I think it commands attention not so much for its large size and effective naturalism but more so because Fildes captured a human relation that is of time immemorial, and we respond instinctively to his depiction of this relation. The painting is a*

powerful image of my own philosophy of medicine—not the posture of a
helpless physian watching the relentless scourge of nature, but the physi-
cian as empathetic witness.

So, all this having been said, how might we situate medical ethics, or more
specifically, how might we ground the particular requirements of a medical
ethics in its broader philosophy? This question, by the parameters drawn
here, becomes: How would medical philosophy appear if it were *based*, à
la Levinas, in Ethics, rather than, let us say, Truth? Concerning the relation
of ethics to epistemology and for that matter, to metaphysics, one might
recall the game children play—"rock, paper, scissors." Simultaneously,
two players throw out a fist, a flat hand or two fingers. The fist, symbolizing
a rock, breaks the scissors, represented by two fingers, but paper, the flat
hand, covers the rock; note however that the scissors cut the paper. Neither
rock, paper, nor scissors is inherently superior to all of the others: Each has
its relation to its counterparts. Analogously, we can explore the position of
ethics relative to the other domains of philosophy of medicine. An ambi-
tious—and, it seems to me, worthwhile—project is to examine a philosophy of medicine based not on its epistemology, but instead on ethics. Simply
put, one might consider the case of ethics prior to truth and its consequences for a philosophy of medicine.

One might reasonably ask, Well, what are the practical implications of
such a philosophical turn? If this proposal frames how we need to in general
foster the humane interaction of health care provider and patient, how
might such specialized medical ethics problems as human experimentation,
care for the dying, guidelines for reproduction technology, and the like,
be affected? The validity of my approach must be tested in such particular
issues, but recall in the previous chapter (pp. 81–82) how we distinguished
two categories of medical ethics: (1) applied ethics, which collects tributaries from jurisprudence, political decision-making, social mores, economic concerns, as well as moral philosophy, and (2) foundational ethical
philosophy, which formulates ethics in a top-down fashion from certain
principles. It is this latter approach that I have adopted. The relational
philosophy outlined here, I argue, should serve as a basis of all medical
practice, for the need to raise moral consciousness seems to me our highest
priority, as we recognize that the doctor-patient relationship is in most

dire jeopardy. It is on this point that my argument must stand. If we can make explicit the unique moral character of the healer, then, I expect, the particular clinical problems calling for moral adjudication will be clarified.

So, rather than become embroiled in particular case examples like doctor-assisted suicide, for instance, I would rather ask the foundational question: Is medical ethics—in the form I am advocating—to remain ancillary to medical education and practice, or can it be moved to center stage? After all, medical ethics, even in its applied form, is hardly a pillar of contemporary medical education. As we have seen, the erosion of a primary concern with a humane ethics can be traced to the end of the nineteenth century, when physiology and its close cousin, medicine, rode upon the broad shoulders of newly defined positivist principles. This new standard of knowledge was to apply an objective natural science to physiology and health; the observer would distance himself as far as possible from the object of scrutiny. As discussed in chapter 1, the dramatic change in American medical education at the turn of the century was presented by the medical establishment as a struggle of a new reductionist ideal of a laboratory-based medicine against an older, descriptive, nonscientific medicine. University-based medical education dominated and then largely extinguished clinical competitors (homeopaths, chiropractors, herbalists, and other "folk" practitioners). The consequences of this revolution have been conceptually far-reaching, the moral implications perhaps unexpected. But we can still correct our course, despite the strength of the underlying positivist ethos.

The prevailing positivist approach need not deny the legitimacy of the interpersonal relation, but in practice it too often subordinates it to laboratory-derived facts. Perhaps a better way of regarding the problem is to say that physicians at times seem to become preoccupied with their scientific persona. They must be reminded that although they are in some sense *like* scientists, this does not mean that they *are* (only) scientists. The moral character of doctoring is something else. It is this "something else" which must be made self-evident. To posit an ethical metaphysics for medicine is no less than to claim that the very foundation of medicine lies in its finding and asserting its own philosophy, a philosophy that I claim should be based on relational ethics.

If the doctor-patient relationship is constructed according to the ethical model outlined here, it markedly alters the approach employed by the physician-scientist. If the patient does not reside in the protected enclave of this relational interaction, he or she is but another object of biological inquiry; and when an illness is divorced from the sufferer in this fashion, the experience of disease is profoundly negatively affected. The objectification of illness as "disease"—as an "object of inquiry"—alienates the individual from his or her body. In illness, the body is experienced in a fundamentally different manner than in everyday life, where we are, for the most part, unaware of our bodies as our medium of experience. But when ill, we not only become aware of pain or dysfunction, but we also attempt to find "meaning" by objectifying the body. I find myself scrutinizing the diseased element as somehow separate from self, outside my identity. The mind-body duality that pervades Western thinking about what it is to be human is nowhere better exhibited than in the case of illness.

The physician is of course party to this process of objectification as he or she attempts to define the disease scientifically by physico-chemical measures. But *I am not* a confluence of blood counts, liver enzyme levels, mineral concentrations, and the like. A radical positivist point of view regards the patient only as a composite of the objective data, and while I recognize that these tests reflect my biochemical nature, the laboratory results are something foreign to my inner sense of personhood. What does it mean to *me* that my calcium is low or high? This process of separating my bodily functions from my intimate experience is the alienation intrinsic to the experience of illness. From this orientation, important distinctions are made between apprehending the body in "lived experience" (i.e., normal, everyday) as opposed to the disruption initiated by illness and its care.

There are strategies for better dealing with this dehumanizing process, and unsurprisingly the best solutions are also, in the everyday sense, the easiest. Health care providers have to listen, respond, and generally account for the subjective experience of a patient's complaint. So much of our discontent can be traced back to the too little time the physician spends with a client, and how poorly a true dialogue develops. Focusing upon the clinical narrative, the patient's rendition of the disease experience offers crucial insight to the physician, both as scientist and empathetic, that is, ethical, healer. Beyond obtaining information that may be important in tending to the patient's particular medical needs, a patient's own description of the illness presents the physician with the problem of suffering, with the profound disruption, uncertainty, and pain that disease imposes. To ignore this aspect of illness is to deny the patients' fundamental humanity and relegate them to the status of object. Only a relational construct, deliberately and carefully effected, can counteract this attitude.

A Relational Approach to Medical Ethics

Resuscitation—the very word elicits panic. Of course physicians and nurses don't panic. They rush about, pound on the chest, administer drugs, breathe for the patient. I stood back recently to watch such an episode in the ICU. There a "code" is rather standard and thus the event was highly coordinated; each role was clearly followed and there was no emotional element that would lead one to believe that the object of this exercise, still on the cusp of life, might as easily fall into oblivion as rejoin her family waiting anxiously outside. If there were any emotions, the veteran lifesavers gave no indication of them. This was only another in a long series of cardiac arrests, the dramatic but rather neutral term for brink-of-death.

My mother arrested, in my home. She had the brass school bell next to her bed to ring if she needed us. She had been sick for a long time, and we were attuned to her 2:00 A.M. asthma attacks, those seemingly intractable episodes where she sat, slightly hunched over, using her neck and chest muscles to inhale just a little more air. The glassy eyes and forlorn, frightened glance she would cast us as she gasped for air announced that the medication was not working. One night, as we rushed in, she gave me one quick look and fell over. She stopped breathing. I cannot recount exactly what happened, but I "resuscitated" her, and when the firemen and ambulance arrived they intubated her, administered oxygen, started an I.V. We drove off to the hospital.

The doctors and nurses were quite impressed with my single-handed feat. I tried to explain that it was nothing like their code, that what I had done, I did in near panic. I could not recall a single detail of my actions after she stopped breathing, nor could I explain why she resumed. All I knew was that when the firemen arrived, she was still alive. My mother lived for another few years, alone, no one available to pull her back from the cusp of the final order. I wasn't there, but I know exactly how she must have experienced her last moments. In a sense, indeed I was there. I had finally experienced death.

At age forty, I began to disengage from science, to study philosophy seriously, and to appeal consciously to my kinder self. No doubt, I am a better doctor. My mother's death had reawakened my initial calling and reminded me that we cannot know our own death, only those of others. In that witness we see ourselves.

Philosophically, we might regard sickness as a disjunction between body (i.e., disease) and mind (i.e., subjectivity). As with all such dualities, part of our dilemma is how to construct a coordinated approach that can reunite both aspects of our identity. In the medical context, the mind/body split is perhaps useful for a scientific approach, but curing illness is not exclusively an epistemological problem. Psychologically, illness as *experience* is deeply invasive of our very integrity as selves, and this becomes a moral problem because *person* is a moral category. The paramount project then becomes one of unification. Rather than dealing with only the fragmentary disease (epistemologically), the physician must address the full person (ethically). In short, we must create the space in a "medical problem" for an ethical solution: The doctor-patient encounter requires a relational philosophy.

Note, please, that this encounter is not one of physician and patient meeting as friends, both dedicated to the good of health. This stance is referred to as "beneficence"—mutual sympathy in the interest and the common pursuit of health. Such a relationship assumes that the doctor and patient share the same medical ideals, have no conflicting economic or social interests, and embrace the same moral values. These are of course broad, and too often unwarranted, assumptions. An ethics based on beneficence must seek to establish a common social ground, and more specifically, must build from the complexity of agreeing upon a common goal. The position I am advocating has a very different structure. One might say that relational ethics is in a sense simpler: Rather than having two parties agree on a common goal, the approach begins at an earlier step, namely, when the physician serves the patient as an act of responsibility. There need be no negotiation of what is good or how to reach a particular goal. In this schema, care is an *a priori* ethical relationship; the goals follow.

The physician-patient encounter in the philosophy I have advocated is fundamentally ethical: No contingencies and no caveats. The *unconditional* relationship alone is the *sine qua non* of medicine. So in this respect, interrelational ethics shifts the medical ethics playing field. Beneficence is obviously a guiding principle in the physician-patient encounter, but it is merely a product of the primary relational commitment. Beneficence is the result of a more fundamental ethical mandate. In short, beneficence cannot serve as the defining standard of care.

Finally, when alterity *defines* relationship, the autonomous self is left behind. Autonomy has vanished from the ethical algebra just as beneficence has become a product of the equation. Autonomy shifts from an ideal of self-sufficiency to become a principle of amorality. Although stated quite starkly, this fairly illustrates the divide between a relational and an autonomous ethic. The metaphysical structure of these positions could hardly be more polarized.

So how might one begin to sketch in a philosophy of medicine in this framework? There are three basic precepts.

(1)   The physician-patient relation is already given, *a priori,* as one of responsibility, and this sense of responsibility must emanate from compassion. Thus the health care provider makes a personal commitment, an empathetic product of his or her personality, to the patient. We find this precept in the writings of Hippocrates, and it is present in diverse descriptions of the good physician throughout the ages. In previous eras, when religious consciousness was more freely expressed, we read testaments of this character as love. For instance, Savonarola, a fifteenth-century Dominican visionary, wrote:

The physician that bringeth love and charity to the sick, if he be good and kind and learned and skillful, none can be better than he. Love teacheth him everything, and will be the measure and rule of all the measures and rules of medicine.

In our more secularized times, we base such empathy on what Nathaniel Hawthorne in *The Scarlet Letter* described as some kind of shared intuition:

If the [physician] possess native sagacity, and a nameless something more—let us call it intuition; if he show no intrusive egoism, nor disagreeably prominent characteristics of his own; if he have the power, which must be born in him, to bring his mind into such affinity with his patient's . . . then, at some inevitable moment, will the soul of the sufferer be dissolved, and flow forth in a dark, but transparent stream, bringing all its mysteries into the daylight.

In both passages, the doctor-patient relationship is described as being based on a shared understanding of illness. The doctor does not solely serve as an objective observer, but partakes in a communion with the ill. Responsibility requires a personal *response*, one originating from the deepest recesses of the soul.

One of the most eloquent modern testaments to this relationship is the portrait of an English country doctor, John Sassall, described by John Berger in *A Fortunate Man* (1967). When describing the nature of illness, Berger emphasizes the sufferer's sense of alienation. Dr. Sassall's primary commitment is to revive lost individuality, which he accomplishes through the same process of response and recognition that Levinas described. Berger writes,

Clearly the task of the doctor—unless he merely accepts the illness on its face value and incidentally guarantees for himself a "difficult" patient—is to recognize the man. If the man can begin to feel recognized—and such recognition may well include aspects of his character which he has not recognized himself—the hopeless nature of his unhappiness will have changed. . . .

In sketching the deeply personal encounter of patient and physician, Berger emphasizes the act of recognition, a word he uses repeatedly and deliberately to capture the ethical meeting place. The process of reintegration—healing—requires that the doctor project himself as a comparable person in whom the patient recognizes, despite his aggravated self-consciousness, aspects of him- or herself.

It is the doctor's acceptance of what the patient tells him and the accuracy of his appreciation as he suggests how different parts of his life may fit together, it is this which then persuades the patient that he and the doctor and other men are comparable because whatever he says of himself or his fears or his fantasies seem to be at least as familiar to the doctor as to him. He is no longer an exception. *He can be recognized.* And this is the prerequisite for cure or adaptation. [emphasis added]

Sassall's success hinges upon the "deep but unformulated expectation of the sick for a sense of fraternity. He recognizes them." This is the ethical dimension that informs his practice. He has not forfeited his technical expertise; after all he was a competent surgeon, obstetrician, pediatrician, and internist. But Sassall clearly depended more on his inner ethical muse when dealing with patients than the ability to hide behind his professional, technical persona. He expressed this humane voice in many ways, but I particularly like the following admission:

> Common sense has been a dirty word with me for many years now—except perhaps when it is applied to very factual and easily assessed problems. When dealing with human beings it is my biggest enemy—and tempter. It tempts me to accept the obvious, the easiest, the most readily available answer. It has failed me on almost every occasion I have used it—and God knows how often I have fallen and still fall for the trap.

His chronicler comments, "his satisfaction comes mostly from those cases where he faces forces which no previous explanation will exactly fit, because they depend upon the history of a patient's particular personality. He tries to keep that personality company in its loneliness."

Without prioritizing empathy, we doom ourselves to a myopic technocratic medicine. This is not to say that there is no place for the highly technical solution to certain problems. We have come to expect no less. But this is not an either/or selection. Why not demand humane *and* scientifically competent care? Beyond technical expertise and performance, medical ethics must face perhaps the more difficult challenge of establishing the physician's identification with the patient. This relationship, I maintain, will appropriately position the health care provider as the patient's champion. In the world of managed care, such advocacy will increasingly need to become the physician's role.

(2)   Our medical ethics must acknowledge the primacy of trust, wherein the patient abdicates a significant portion of his or her autonomy. Physicians are trained, and appropriately so, to master extraordinarily complex activities. To perform brain or cardiac surgery is a prodigious intellectual and technical feat; to treat acute leukemia or AIDS requires an enormous fund of knowledge, clinical experience, and judgment. Patients immediately forfeit their autonomous status solely on the basis of this gulf in knowledge. Judgment is the crucial ingredient, and when we are sick, we lose our capacity for objectivity. In this dependence, grades of freedom have necessarily been forfeited. The relation between equals in the original

Levinasian scheme has lost its parity. The equation has assumed a new complexity and the casualty is patient autonomy, so much the subject of recent bioethics.

"How's Dr. Cassidy?"

"Well, you know, he's 89. He just couldn't tolerate the full dose of chemotherapy."

"What? Why did you give him full dose?!"

"Hmm . . . He insisted."

"That's ridiculous. Who's the doctor, anyway?"

"Me, obviously. Give me a break! You know he's treated more lymphoma cases than the entire staff put together. I deferred to him this time. The next round, he gets half dose."

"Yeah, if he survives the first."

The autonomy question is highly problematic, and I believe the real issue is defining professional trust. On the one hand, we want to control our destiny, but more often than not we must forfeit the opportunity and obligation of making choices. Medical decisions are made for us. At the same time, mistakes are made, even by informed patients and well-meaning physicians. Our innocence of the future denies our doing anything with complete confidence. When the doctor recites a statistic that a particular therapy offers an 80 percent likelihood for cure, what is the relevance for an individual patient? There is a one chance in five that the therapy will fail, and only the trial will determine the outcome in the particular case. We must make the best informed choice, but that choice is never guaranteed to be correct. There are many unknowable factors at play, and the statistics can only inform and direct our choice, for they are descriptive, and only partially so. This is an important distinction. We try to pick the best option, but often we do not know what that might be. We endeavor to anticipate consequences with intelligent (i.e. rationally based) guesses and hope for the best.

To deal with uncertainty, professional judgement and extensive experience are required. Trust in the physician thus naturally erodes patient autonomy within the context of illness. Patients need to be informed, they must be free to make choices, and they are ultimately responsible for accepting medical risks; but these are qualified degrees of autonomy. The patient ultimately relies on the health professional for guidance. I am not advocating paternalism, but autonomy thus viewed does lose much of its sacrosanct character. Stated starkly, autonomy has a subordinate status in my description of medicine's ethical universe.

(3)   Although I have argued for a relational ethics, this construction cannot be based on a Levinasian formulation, where there is a reciprocal relationship between Self and Other (i.e., where the Self is defined by the Other in the relational equation, and the Other is also a self, defined reciprocally). In medicine, the equation between Self and Other is categorically nonsymmetrical. The requirement that the patient must trust the physician's ability hardly allows for reciprocity. Now as I attempt to describe medical ethics as an application of such a relational philosophy, I must acknowledge that the engagement of Self and Other no longer possesses the equality of free encounter. Specifically, when we consider the position of the patient, we see that the power of the relational construct is most aptly applied as a vector from the physician toward the patient. The reverse is encumbered by dependence. The issue of restoring the patient's full sense of personhood might be construed as uncomfortably passive in this scheme. But the physician as healer ethically commits herself to reestablishing the sufferer's complete identity. The relationship may not be symmetrical as the sufferer suffers, but the *goal* of healing is in fact to affirm an equal exchange between full selves. The healer's success is in the patient again becoming his true self, but the equation is not solely one-sided either. By establishing an empathetic identification with the patient, in truly *seeing* the patient, the professional experiences herself. Thus the task of medical ethics centered on the clinician-patient encounter actualizes both patient and healer. Each becomes a *relational* self.

By posing the issues in this fashion I have attempted to present explicitly what I perceive to be the essential problem in philosophy of medicine, or more to the point, *the* problem of medicine, which so poignantly and dramatically exhibits the very issue of postmodern selves in a postmodern world. We seek to ground a moral view while respecting different beliefs and cultural demands and thus protecting the Other from becoming an object. And the other side of the ledger is also delineated. Ultimately, the clinician is defined through care and responsibility, emerging into an ethical space resplendent with the opportunity to become true selves. After all, this must be regarded as the fulfillment of his professional aspirations.

Medicine is a unique crucible in which to test these precepts. If philosophy is to help us understand who we are and how we order and engage the world, I see the ethical component not as an attachment, but as the foundation of clinical practice. At this locus medicine is naturally situated. So when we ask, "What is medicine?" I would begin with "Medicine is ethical." The rest then follows.

6

Metaphysical Musings

The Infinite Beckons

Medicine as a clinical activity always fascinated me, awed me. I still have not lost my sense of wonder at the sheer power of the medical encounter. But my appreciation has evolved over time.

There are many memories of those first patients I met during medical school. Although I trained in Boston, my clinical introduction was at the Mayo Clinic. My father, who thought the Mayo was humanity's ultimate triumph, had arranged for me to do a third-year medical student clerkship at the hospital there. It was a unique institution in my experience. A huge medical complex, with literally thousands of patients processed in the out-patient clinics and a significant percentage of them hospitalized under various sub-specialty services. I was very impressed with the efficiency and the richness of the pathology passing daily through its venerable doors. Assigned to the gastroenterology service, I found myself in the train of residents and fellows following the staff physician every day on his rounds. He was a knowledgeable doctor, with a British accent that conferred another dimension of authority. He carried his responsibilities with a certain air appropriate to his station.

I learned a lot that summer, but my starkest memory had nothing to do with scientific or clinical knowledge. The team was visiting a woman in her thirties; she had straw blond hair, a waxy complexion, and shrunken eyes. Emaciated and frightened, she was one of those typical midwestern working women who flocked to the Mayo Clinic as a medical mecca, and in retrospect I can better understand her complete bafflement when Dr. English intoned, "My dear lady, I am sorry to say that you have cancer of the pancreas. There is nothing we can do for you. You will simply have to get used to the idea that you will soon die. I'm not sure when, but if I were you, I would put my things in order. You will be discharged tomorrow." And with that, he turned abruptly and his entourage followed. For a moment I was immobilized in utter amazement. I could not believe the scene I had just witnessed, nor could I respond. I lowered my head and followed my colleagues. Thus began my induction into the medical fraternity.

When I returned to Boston and began my internal medicine rotation at the Boston City Hospital, I was well prepared for the demands of the resident-run medical wards. Now this was fun. With apparent independence, the residents decided diagnostic procedures, therapies, disposition issues—in fact, they were in charge. Unlike the Mayo Clinic, there was an informality, a camaraderie that could only emerge from the cohesiveness of a fighting unit engaged in trench warfare. We were in the pits of a strapped municipal hospital, saving the down-trodden from their alcoholism, drug addiction, trauma, infections, diabetes, heart disease. When some returned regularly, we welcomed them back like old friends to a safe haven. Pneumonia was a small price to pay to escape mean streets.

By the end of two months I was functioning as an intern, and the more desperate the patient, the sicker he or she might be, the more excited I became. My triumph in that period was the discovery that Mr. Antonio Desmarais, covered with lice and feces, suffering acute alcohol withdrawal with delirium tremens, also had pulmonary tuberculosis. I, after four other students, interns, and residents had failed to discover the faint pink bacillus, pointed one out to them all. I was convinced that it was the victory of an acute eye, an active intelligence, and an untiring rigor. In fact it was the thirst for professional approval that drove me relentlessly.

Later I became a resident, and ruled the ward like a drill sergeant. When the chief-of-medicine and I argued whether Mrs. Chafee had pulmonary hypertension, I wheeled her down to the CCU and did a heart catherization. (I was correct in my diagnostic speculations!) When Mr. Pearlmutter was declared brain dead, I informed the family and literally pulled the plug. When our next door neighbor slit his wrists in a sexual debauch, I detachedly marveled at his tendons, explaining how they exactly followed the depiction in my anatomy textbook, and then unceremoniously

*drove him to the emergency room. I delighted in my knowledge and my
authority.*

*I also assumed a particular ethical stance regarding patient care, which
I haughtily regarded as dispassionately honest. I never played the game.
The game, or at least the theatrics by which I then termed it, was to offer
the patient a potentially false sense of hope, to give misplaced confidence
that an answer was forthcoming, or the desired assurance that a therapy
would be successful. I remained in many respects aloof, afraid of misrepre-
senting either myself or what medicine might offer. The patient's craving
for such support was relegated to another, perhaps a nurse—they were
generally nurturing; psychiatrists or ministers might help—it was after all
their job. I was strictly business, an entrepreneur of positivism, a budding
scientist, a man of the world of facts. I was a brash, arrogant technocrat—
a young prince of the dominion, full of the power at my command.*

Medicine may be viewed as a moral microcosm. We admire physicians not
only because they have technical expertise, but also because their knowledge can save and enrich life. In this sense the health care provider is
informed and oriented by an ethical mandate. We might be satisfied with
the apparent value of medicine's agenda of promoting life and leave our
examination of the roots of medical ethics at this point. I think that is a
fair place to stop, but I dare not. The value we attribute to life is not
necessarily shared by all cultures, and I suspect that our preoccupation with
health reflects an elusive metaphysical view of the world and ourselves. It
may seem hopeless to attempt an examination of issues so deeply embedded, if not hidden, but I feel compelled to do so, because we have yet to
exhaust the potential enrichment and erudition offered by the concepts of
two philosophers discussed earlier. The first is Nietzsche's idea of eternal
recurrence, and the second, Levinas's formulation of the Other as constitutive of ourselves. Although I proceed in this direction, I do so with some
hesitation. Each presents an avenue of approach to the questions which
persistently haunt me, but this is territory pocked with obstacles and deep
holes. Their presentations are frankly metaphysical, and whether I walk
there as a physician-scientist or as a philosopher, metaphysics is dangerous
ground. But ethics emanates from metaphysics—from after physics, from

beyond empirical knowledge. To proceed with this project I must engage the question of *why* our encounter with the Other demands a moral response. Why indeed should I respond generously? To what call do I harken? Nietzsche and Levinas, different in their respective ethics, nonetheless display an interesting commonality in their responses to the infinite, and so provide a metaphysical answer. We should listen.

Eternal Recurrence

Nietzsche was a pivotal critic of the Judeo-Christian tradition of ethics, arguing instead for a morality that had neither revealed status, nor universal standing, nor philosophical foundation—to wit, no ethical imperative. He may also be regarded as the "last metaphysician" (as Martin Heidegger characterized him), for even though Nietzsche attacked an older theology, his philosophy nonetheless sought to achieve a metaphysical truth by which moral action could be guided. We have already considered the nature of the moral agent as the hero striving for autonomous self-aggrandizement, but what ethics beyond self-fulfillment of such a Darwinian animal guides us? The "answer"—decidedly postmodern because of its indeterminant character—resides in a nebulous metaphysical appreciation of our place in time. For Nietzsche, like all great metaphysicians, regards our *place*—that by which we are "situated" and thus oriented to *know*—in the even more elusive, yet fundamental, temporality of nature. To appreciate ourselves in time is to bestow meaning on our unknowing biological character. It is here that he would hope to describe a moral philosophy.

Nietzsche's philosophy achieves its most profound metaphysical depths in what he called *eternal recurrence*. Eternal recurrence, like Nietzsche's conception of Man, is fundamentally organic, a description of life as renewal, regeneration, and return. I believe Nietzsche uses eternal recurrence not as a theory of the world, but of the self. The notion of eternal recurrence fuses Nietzsche's concepts of the Will to Power and its corollary, *becoming* as true being. We are enjoined to live as if each moment is to be relived, unchanged, into eternity. The eternal recurrence is the final destination of a deeply rooted evolutionary process, a calling that should become an ethic of our biological being, independent of any transcendent principle. With that perspective, each moment is not only immutable, but precious, making us forever accountable to ourselves. Nietzsche's recurrence does not refer to a life precisely *like* this one, but to this *very same* life. He would thus imbue the quality of eternity into every moment, and lead us to a supreme self-awareness of our ultimate and inescapable responsibility for our acts. The last element of his ethics, then, is to accept the irrevocability of every choice and thereby allow us to assume the mandate of responsibility for our life, a life to be lived again and again, eternally.

If God is dead, then our morality must be based on our self-willed sovereignty. Responsibility then resides solely in the individual, whose identity is based on fully acknowledging the primacy of the will to power and living its mandate freed of false and encumbering moral restrictions. This is a commitment only the strong can assume, for the sick sigh (as he wrote in *On the Genealogy of Morals*), "If only I were someone else." If life is to be eternally recurrent, then we must accept living in the present in its full and self-sufficient complement. Time is framed not in the past or future, but it accompanies us, moving steadily forward within the present.

The will, alone on its own axis, unselfconsciously knows no past or future. Eternal recurrence, as an *ethical* mandate, becomes the ultimate assertion of that will. It is precisely the elevation of man the animal from the one-dimensional will to a second ethical dimension that allows a moral exercise of will to alter the self, and thereby let it become freed and healed. The power of the eternal recurrence can be seen in its full expression when the past is altered by the will in the present. The present vision of the self thus defines the past, and if the present is accepted, then all that has led to that juncture has been enjoined. Most important, the past has formed the future. Thus to accept the present in Nietzsche's terms is to have willed— or willed to choose to accept—all that led to this moment. Here then is an expansive ethical view, in which a fully creative will is celebrated and redemption may be thus attained.

The moral structure of eternal recurrence is that we must live each moment as if it is to recur again and again into eternity. To suffer the effects of lassitude, weakness, distraction, or debility into the infinite expanse of time is truly a moral consequence of overwhelming significance. The thought evokes a frightening descent into hell. But I suspect that Nietzsche was far more concerned to inspire an awareness of our present predicament so that we acknowledge that we must seek a point of orientation outside ourselves and our normal experience—a metaphysical orientation. (Let me again note that contemporary analytical philosophy disallows attaining such an Archimedean perspective, and perhaps this is the most acute separation between the analytical and metaphysical points of view. I self-consciously step out of the analytical tradition into the older metaphysical one in order to initiate a discussion of these moral questions.)

Ironically, Nietzsche, who pronounced God dead, was a great metaphysician who sought a solution in ethics, the domain most intimately identified with being human—all too human. *Eternal recurrence is a metaphor for responsibility.* From where does that responsibility arise? It must come from an appreciation of our place in the universe as one small instant in time and space occupied by a minute consciousness that nonetheless recognizes—to whatever limited extent—our niche in the infinite. As I have already discussed regarding Levinas's notions of reflexivity, recognizing our very existence is *the* act of self-consciousness. With that recognition, we enter into a stream of time that knows neither beginning nor end.

This metaphysical domain becomes moral when we perceive that we must—and do—act in an infinite cosmos, whose entire meaning rests upon the fact that we confer it. *We* confer the value of existence, and despite our infinitesimally puny place in the universe, our accord is its basis of meaning. *We* create meaning. Meaning is metaphysical. And meaning is moral.

The Face

Levinas takes us to the same place by a different road. He, like Nietzsche, seeks a vehicle by which we might orient ourselves metaphysically, that is to say, by a point beyond ourselves. On his view, recognizing that we are individuals requires that we separate ourselves from the everyday world. This is the preliminary step toward delineating the finite from the infinite. Separated man or woman is no longer one with the totality of being, but is turned out to face the infinite. Here, in the knowledge that the world and we ourselves are situated in an infinity of space and time is to acknowledge that we have encountered, engaged, recognized a fathomless "not-I."

How is the infinite perceived? Wittgenstein maintained that there is nothing to be said about such things. What is metaphysical is beyond rationality, beyond language, beyond description. He might acknowledge its being, but he could entertain no further comment. Levinas, however, seeks to express this most profound experience and he depicts it by describing how the isolated self, when interrupted by another, is extroverted—turned outward to face "infinity," to face that which cannot be known. The Self confronts the infinite through the recognition of the Other, which resides in a radically different domain. Thus the infinite is sensed in the *face* of an Other. In that encounter there is both the presentation of vulnerability of that face and the astonishment of its incomprehensibility. The face thus becomes a window to the infinite.

The encounter with the face eclipses the finite—the particular, circumscribed totality, our everyday lives—as lived nonreflectively. More than framing the response, the encounter also actualizes the self. In other words, the Self is in its very essence reflexive, aware of itself as a self, as a person within a context in which it acts, thinks, remembers, and feels. In this view, to be a self is to be self-aware of one's identity in a world where identity is not given, but must be created and formed against or with others. To be self-contained, or self-sufficient—to exist nonreflexively—is to be unaware of one's place in the world, and more specifically to either ignore or deny the infinite. The face of the other challenges this complacency. Not to be ranked as a modality of coexistence (a sociological issue), nor even of knowledge (an epistemological project), the face becomes "the primordial production of being" (a metaphysics). We might only "approach" or "intend" the infinite, but in that effort, we truly realize our own selfhood.

Herein lies an ethical metaphysics. The face, a concrete expression of the infinite, enables us to recognize the limits of our experience as totality. "Totality" is used ironically; we are not true Selves until we face the infinite. This is the same metaphysical posture Nietzsche assumes with eternal recurrence: to recognize the import of the infinite is to reveal our deepest metaphysical yearnings. For Levinas, the face of the other, or more specifically the encounter with that face, is our conduit to the infinite, and in its demand for response, a moral space is created—the locus of the possibility of all those expressions that are the basis of a moral life. Perhaps it is useful to think that to face the infinite is to confront our ethical possibilities, filling the "content" of a person's view of the world.

As we recognize the Other, the infinite, the non-Self, we confront our moral challenge. This idea is not novel to Levinas, but reflects a recurrent metaphysical theme in Western thought, originating at least formally with Augustine, if not integral to the Bible itself. Man cannot be regarded in his complete potential without the inclusion of this fundamental relation to the infinite via the human other. In dialogue, the need to respond evokes responsibility, and it is this response to the Other that finalizes the Self's own reality. This attention to the other is not an actualization of a potential because it is not a potential, not even conceivable, without the other. A relational, responsive ethics becomes our metaphysics.

To Face Ourselves

No man is an island, entire of itself; every man is a piece of the continent, a part of the main . . . any man's death diminishes me, because I am involved in mankind; and therefore never send to know for whom the bell tolls; it tolls for thee.
—*John Donne (1573–1631),* Devotions XVII

We neither assert nor define ourselves without the Other. In this very act of contemplating our "Self," what constitutes ourselves as perceiving and feeling beings, we discover the very basis of our humanity. Thus to separate from our worldly life and face the infinite is the fundamental ethical act. Since the Self does not exist until it confronts the Other—the face, the infinite—one might argue that the Self has been deconstructed, that is, profoundly emptied of "itself." If successful, this formulation has shifted the problem of selfhood that preoccupied our earlier discussion from the Enlightenment project of discerning a knowing entity to one now committed to defining the agency of a moral construct. From here we might erect a contemporary medical ethics.

Because medicine deals so immediately with moral knots, it offers us the powerful occasion in which we may forge the potential of the approach I have advocated. But I must admit in closing an undeclared but implicit theme: While we have concentrated on the clinical setting, this is only a particular case of the vexing general moral conundrum we face in our secular pluralistic society. There are, to be sure, particular issues in medicine that demand attention, and notwithstanding their import, ultimately we seek a strategy by which our humanity might be restored.

I have embraced a relational approach because I believe it effectively addresses our postmodern nihilism by resonating with the well-springs of Western ethics: Biblical communalism and dialogue—inspired by divine address—and the Greek notion of the eternal Good. These fundamental precepts have been refashioned in answer to the philosophical and social critiques peculiar to our own times. We require new metaphors to grope toward a new theory which will allow us to establish the means to transcend our complacency. The face of the Other is a powerful image that directs the discussion to a universal experience, and in the case of medicine, I can think of no better vehicle to carry these complex and often freighted issues.

But there is a second, perhaps more obscure agenda hidden beneath this discussion of the ethical foundations of medicine, translated as the service function of the clinician. We have dealt almost exclusively with the ethical concerns for others, but now I want to direct attention to how the health care provider is fulfilled by his or her professional duties, and how the moral realization translates into personal gratification. Altruism has an intrinsic contradiction gnawing at its character: Often, we suspect the charitable or empathetic act as truly fulfilling the giver's need to give, completing his or her own psychological desires. Thus the altruist may be viewed as ultimately selfish. Does this interpretation somehow dampen or restrict the moral act? Hardly. It seems clear to me that by recognizing motive we have only gained some insight into the sources of the energy driving certain behavior. The act itself remains untarnished. But we do find interesting consequences if we examine the moral act from the *agent's* perspective, and in doing so I hope to reveal the rich metaphysical dimensions of the caring act. Responsibility entails self-fulfillment. By assuming responsibility for care, the doctor or nurse is "actualized," which is a fancy way of saying that in enacting the professional mandate the individual completes his or her chosen identity.

I have avoided until now the distinctive roles of physician and nurse, and I have assumed each under a common banner—"the health care provider." In fact, there are important distinctions, especially germane for this discussion. In the era I was trained, doctors assumed an authority—and dominance—that largely precluded a decision-making function for the nurse. That dichotomy has been weakened in the past decade, and nurses now assume expanded responsibility in the care of the patient. For instance, in one of Boston's most prestigious teaching hospitals, nurses are encouraged to seek independent medical consultations if they perceive that the interests of their patients might be better served. But I am not simply referring to nurse practitioners who function as surrogate physicians, or nurse administrators who have increasingly played a part in health care administration, but rather to nurses who still occupy their traditional place in the setting of patient care in the clinic or hospital ward, where they generally have a more direct and comprehensive role in caring for the patient than the physician does. My philosophical discussion is thus most directly pointed to the physician who has to overcome a duality governed by two distinctive ethics. It is the struggle between them that has given us the most direct insight into medicine's current structure.

Doctors assume two functions simultaneously: On the one hand, they are like colonels in the army, directing immediate troop movements and devising future strategy; on the other, they also function at times as foot soldiers, assuming patients' burdens by advising and consoling them, performing procedures on their bodies, and other such acts that are both intimate and personally engaging. Nursing, by and large, has no such duality, and even in today's large hospitals and clinics, the nurses' care of the patient is essentially intimate, despite their expanding administrative roles. In the very act of personalized attention, the nurse has few responsibilities that compete with these private acts, which constitute the primary interpersonal encounter. To the extent that nurses distance themselves from the patient, we are struck by the discordance of that failed amity.

We were at dinner, talking about the children, politics, work. The conversation drifted to the issues I was grappling with in writing this book, and I observed how nurses really took care of patients and doctors too often suffered—or enjoyed—a certain distance from them. Cheryl immediately picked up the theme and commented:

"I had my first baby in San Bernadino. The delivery itself was grueling— 36 hours of labor, then a C-section—but the total experience was wonderful, not least of all because the nurses were just terrific. Post-op, I was flattened, and they cared for me, discussed what we should name the baby, cooed over her and encouraged me. They really turned something that in so many ways was so traumatic into a very special, wonderful time.

"So I was totally unprepared for what awaited me in New York. Exactly two years later, very pregnant with my second baby, I toured the hospital where I was to give birth to Shelly. What I saw in the nursery made me heartsick. The nurses handled the babies like they were pieces of meat. I sensed no care, no nurturing—in fact, I was stunned by their hostility. Before I left, I made sure that I had signed all the necessary paperwork to keep my baby with me at all times in my room. I wanted nothing to do with that nursery.

"My time came; I labored, this time only for five hours, and then my doctor delivered my second daughter surgically. Several hours after her birth, I woke up to see one of the nurses wheeling her out of my room. 'Excuse me. Please bring her back. I have rooming-in privileges.' Opening the door without breaking her stride, the nurse calmly said, 'Well, you're sleeping, and she has to be changed. I change them in the nursery.'

"Striving to control my alarm, I proposed (there were diapers galore in my nightstand) that she change her in the room. 'No.' 'Well, I really don't want her away from me.' With that, the nurse snapped the door shut, abruptly wheeled Shelly back to my side, strode away and called back, 'Then you change her.' 'But I can't move—I've just had a section' (did she really not know?). 'You want the staff to change her, she goes to the nursery.' And with that she left.

"So that was the first diaper of my second baby. Shaking in frustration and anger, still incredulous, too hurt from the incision to move much at all, tears streaming, I changed that goddamn diaper somehow. The nurses never voluntarily touched her again. That evening when my husband came to visit us, I told him, 'You've got to get us out of here as quickly as possible.' And I put a phone call into my physician, telling him what had happened.

"This began the open warfare between the nurses and me. The pain medication never showed up on time; no one was ever there to lift Shelly to me; the water pitcher remained mysteriously empty. I refused to give them the satisfaction of asking for anything, and somehow stumbled through these minute and impossible chores myself. But then, unfortunately, I needed to have an IV introduced, and I was stuck. I requested a doctor. Impossible. The nurse would do it.

*"I extended my left hand. She jabbed me once. I looked her right in the
eyes; she never lifted hers. Face studiously neutral, she jabbed me again. No
go. Again. The veins were prominent; I'd never had this problem before. I
continued to stare at her, and then uncontrollably began to question her
even as, equally uncontrollably, I shook and wept with rage. 'HOW can
you do this? HOW can you call yourself a nurse and act this way? Don't
you think I know what you're doing? How can you act this way?' again
and again. She would not look at me; but, finally, the needle did get properly located. Silent, controlled, she finished her business and left the room.*

*"My doctor was the very best of the three different OBs I had for my
different deliveries. But because of those nurses, that delivery was a night-
mare, the worst."*

"So Cheryl, why?"

*"Don't get me started. I have my suspicions, but I don't know. Does it
matter?"*

"No, of course not."

As already discussed, following the Levinasian construct, the very act of
response fulfills the innate potential of the professional's role. But now we
come to an unstated revelation. Beyond the actualization process, where
the selfhood of the physician or nurse becomes fully manifest, there is a
secret cathexis in witnessing, one that occurs in the deepest recesses of
one's soul; namely—speaking as a physician—facing our own selves as an
other. Objectification of disease protects us from the most empathetic
act—confronting ourselves as sufferers, as dying. I am convinced that science, beyond its powerful epistemology, provides a veil, if not a cover, for
the life and death experiences that are so immediately and profoundly
presented to the doctor and nurse by the seriously ill. It is this dimension
of severe suffering and death experienced intimately that deserves final
comment.

This reflection of ourselves as an other can occur under many circumstances. One need not be a witness to disease and the dying to appreciate
this recognition. An important common experience is the confrontation
with our own intimate histories. Our memories conjure up images of ourselves that may seem quite alien to our present state of being. This current
picture may refashion the past to better coincide with our present orienta-

tion, or it may jar us into reassessing ourselves to become more congruent with what we conceive as a more authentic person, frozen as a past image in our memory. In this sense, the memory of our own selves serves as an interior Other that commands attention and response.

But there is another inescapable confrontation we all must face: We become an other when we contemplate our own death. There can be no more finality and finitude to our selfness, no more otherness than our own nonexistence. In medicine, we face the specter of death constantly. Our hospitals have not entirely shed their nineteenth-century aura as houses of death, when to be placed in the infirmary was too often tantamount to a prescription for dying. One does not require a lethal disease to be apprehensive, if not forthrightly frightened. Even today hospitalization is a serious matter, and no procedure, no matter how trivial, can be viewed as inconsequential. Each life setting has risk; hospitals are simply riskier than most other places.

Clinicians—some more than others—face death as a regular feature of work, and like any mortal must deal with the emotional repercussions of witnessing the death of another. For the novice medical or nursing student these first encounters are almost universally difficult emotional experiences. Beyond the sympathy that is evoked, there is an element of voyeurism soon hidden; it hardly comforts the patient to become an object of fascination and wonder, even in the name of science and education. There is a delicate balance between teaching the art of medicine and displaying the patient as some kind of curiosity object. But the fascination remains, because the mystery of death and dying never loses its power. The Self behind the face somehow no longer exists, and as we contemplate the loss of the Other's life our own mortality looms before us. We face infinity—the infinity of nonexistence—most immediately. There is no escape, and whether we see heaven, hell, eternal recurrence, or the void, we recognize our own inevitable termination. Eventually, each of us must join the infinite in one form or another. This is the metaphysical horror of recognizing our true otherness, the end of our being. There is no respite, and those who seek to deny their finitude hide only momentarily from their own fear.

We cannot *know* our own death, but we may see it portended in the throes of another's. We cannot escape the identification. We cannot know our own demise, but can only imagine it as observed in another's. By their example we inevitably ask, Will we expire quickly or in prolonged agony? By accident, by disease, by violence? With loved ones, or alone? Will fear or tranquility rule us in our last moments? Who will mourn and who will not? Is there a soul? Who then am I? Whether we are self-consciously aware or not, our own death looms before us. The infinite beckons and we must respond. In the everyday world, the face of the Other effectively calls us to respond, but it is ultimately only a refraction of our personal otherness. Death is our own mirror.

It was a sunny afternoon. I was returning from apple-picking with the boys. We were cruising back to Boston on Route 2, listening to Marvin Gaye on the radio, laughing at each other's stories, and delighting in the crispness of the day.

As we ascended a gently sloping hill, a car, dark and low to the ground, whisked past us, passing on the right and swerving dangerously into our left lane. I slowed down, and then to my horror saw it smash into another car turning across the highway at the hill's crest.

I braked quickly, pulled over to the shoulder of the road, and ran over to both cars. Out of the reckless car emerged two adolescent boys, who immediately hurled bottles into the woods lining the roadside. In the other car, a man was hunched over the steering wheel. He was moving. His passenger was not.

I quickly examined the young woman. Her side of the car had received the full impact of the crash. She was ashen grey, but I could still appreciate the fine features of her face, her lithe body, her fine clothes. A small line of blood trickled from the corner of her mouth. Her stillness was absolute.

I couldn't open her door. Others appeared and pulled both the driver and his passenger out of the car. She was stretched out on the ground and I examined her quickly. No breathing; no pulse. I put my ear to her chest. No heart sounds. I began mouth-to-mouth resuscitation while someone else pounded her chest. No response. No response.

The paramedics arrived and began their own resuscitation efforts. She was removed to the hospital. I called later. She was dead on arrival: broken neck, severed larynx. She had been a music student, twenty-one years old, engaged to be married to the driver, a lawyer.

That night I was reading Milan Kundera's The Unbearable Lightness of Being, *and was struck by the opening passage of the novel which concerns Nietzsche's eternal recurrence. Kundera wrote, "If eternal return is the heaviest of burdens, then our lives can stand out against it in all their splendid lightness." Kundera's cynicism overwhelmed me. Because we do not believe in eternal recurrence, responsibility eludes us. Everything in this world is pardoned in advance, and therefore everything cynically permitted.*

Several months later I made inquiries about the case. Although I had given my name to the police, I was never contacted. By the time I followed my reborn curiosity, the magistrate had passed judgment. The court officer intoned, "The accident resulted from the confluence of an illegal left hand turn and borderline levels of alcohol intoxication." Penalties were minimal; everyone involved was on probation.

So am I.

Epilogue

"Fred, do you remember Bobby?

"Who?"

"I think his last name was Edwards."

"Dad, I have no idea who you're talking about."

"Sure you do. You must! He was your best friend in third grade."

"Well, I don't. Why do you?"

"Oh, I don't know. Watching Joel run around reminded me of you at that age. I recall how you played ball with Bobby. Don't you remember anything?!"

"Sure, I do . . . "

I remember running down the alley to look at the screaming fire engines. I was no more than two and a half. My memory of eating a chocolate ice cream cone in front of the Georgia Avenue polar bear statue at age three is vivid. I remember pointing out the directions to Granny's at three and a half. I remember first holding my baby sister at age four. I remember the ether mask over my face and the sheer panic of suffocating at four and a half, and the first day of school a few months later. Of those years, I remember my red train engine, the six shooter, the teddy bear, the smell of my room, the wet heat of July nights, the briskness of October, the January snow. I bristle still at the memory of my frustration while waiting for my mother to get off the phone. I remember the illustrated Just So Stories *of Kipling and the unformed excitement I felt looking at the picture of native women standing on a captive's back. I remember my parents listening to the radio and the magic of our first television . . . I remember the tumbling logs falling on my delirious feverish body, the pain in my ear; I remember the tea with milk my mother brought me, and her soothing hand. . . .*

I remember more, much more. But I do not remember Bobby.

We retain what we value, and we know what we want to know or need to know. We forget what we do not use or somehow cannot make part of ourselves. And some memories we want to lose, but cannot. Those are part of our psyche that live in a separate locale—part of us, yet somehow different.

Our memory is selective and intimate. We act in the world, but we are aware of ourselves in large measure through our recollections as we live within ourselves. We feel and we intuit unformed or partially constructed ideas. These occur in the ongoing present. Memory is another function altogether. In ways deeply personal to our most inner being, we rest within ourselves as we recall other personae formed in different contexts of time and place. In our attempts to situate ourselves in those past worlds of childhood, adolescence, young adulthood, middle age, and on, we bring the past with us. We require a construction to enable us to establish a continuous flow of identity between the present and the ever receding past.

Memory is crafted. There is no recall that is not filtered by intervening experience, and that experience interprets and reshapes the original experience. While memory helps to maintain continuity with the past, it too is reshaped to accommodate our present persona. We know, albeit implicitly, that our memory is a critical faculty in shaping our identities. We constantly refashion ourselves to adjust to new demands, goals, ideas, relationships. Our memories are modulated as we redesign our views of ourselves and our world, because memory is so intimate to our very selves.

Memory is a faculty of knowledge. It is highly subjective, private, and untestable without extraordinary effort. To make a memory valid, to test its authenticity, we must perform historical analysis. For instance, who is Bobby Edwards? Was he in fact named Robert Edwards, and was he born as I was in 1947, or was it 1946 or 1948? I could check the birth records of Washington D.C. where we lived when I presumably knew him, but perhaps he was born in Baltimore or Richmond or Dallas. Washington in the 1950s was a migrant town, a sleepy southern city with pretensions to being a major metropolis. Natives were rare. I might go to the elementary school records in search of his demographics. Perhaps a military record would be better. But what if he died in Viet Nam? I would have to find his parents or siblings. There might not be any family left. Forty years ago is a long time to find traces of an everyday sort of guy.

But even if I found traces of this boy, how would I know he had been my best friend? If he is still alive perhaps I could interview him. But if he were famous, perhaps he would not deign to speak with me! Or he might be demented, imprisoned, comatose, or just plain unfriendly. I would have to find him and ask, "Do you remember me?" If he said, "Yes," would I believe him? If he said, "No," what would that prove about our friendship? Only that he too forgot. Or perhaps my father had a faulty memory. Maybe he confused Bobby Edwards with Jimmy Russell; Edwards was in fact the newspaper boy with whom I had no dealings, and Russell was my best friend in the third grade. I could of course determine all of this, but it has no importance to me. Far more significant would be that Kipling book, to look at those pictures again. Would the tied man with native women stomping on his back still excite me? I wonder. Since I remember the picture, I am fairly certain that the old feelings would return. In fact, the mere memory asserts that they would.

We use both history and memory to attempt to capture the past and bring it into the present to better understand ourselves now. We use each to interpret the past in order to interpret the present and, perhaps, to better predict the future. We rely on each to situate ourselves in the confusion of our own time, and to seek the antecedents of our present predicaments and knowledge. These are critical functions to be sure, but memory has another function altogether, also shared by history but less self-consciously. I am referring to memory's essentially moral character.

Memory is moral. I am not referring to "right and wrong" in the normal sense. We do not have right and wrong memories. They may be faulty, mistaken, fantasy, but that is not the issue here. Rather, I am referring to memory as moral in the more general view of human action. How do we regard ourselves as humans, how do we think of a good life, a virtuous act, our interpersonal interactions? These are all moral questions arising from our selves as moral agents. We recognize and incorporate the past into our present lives, as we make the past our own. By doing so, we assume a certain identity. That identity is fundamentally moral in character because it is a judgment about ourselves of who we are and what we hope to be. From that understanding we situate ourselves in the world and act accordingly.

I am not referring to our "psychology," but rather to our moral life. Who we are, what we were and what we hope to be fall squarely in the moral domain. These are evaluative judgments, interpretations of our person. From this perspective the Self is fundamentally a moral category. I would not say that memory cannot also be regarded as a faculty by which we comprehend and order our world. It is certainly part of the mental agency we refer to as "knowing." But what makes memory moral is that we *choose* our recollections, constructing them within a particular framework that has value to us. It is the overriding value-ladenness of memory that radically modulates its status as knowledge. Because memory need not be anything but private, it may safely reflect our most intimate personal values and serve us in living them. We do not, under normal circumstances, attempt to convert our memory into verifiable history, objective (i.e., public) knowledge. We might do so, but generally we are content to believe our memory, for it is about ourselves, and we live with and depend on our subjectivity. In this important way, memory is a means of identifying ourselves.

History is different in this regard because of its public nature. Historians generate common knowledge, and they attempt to do so by scientific methods. Science, ostensibly the epistemological model for all human knowledge, claiming for its method the most independent form of knowing, has strict criteria for acceptable facts and theory. Scientific explanation should be consistent, simple, cohesive, predictive, and as comprehensive as possible. These are highly effective means for obtaining certain kinds of knowledge about the world, and we value these characteristics of scientific information and theory as objective. But objectivity obviously arises from consensus, and standards of consensus are always changing. Criteria of proof have a long history of metamorphosis; assumptions about rationality modify similarly; even Truth can no longer be designated as stable. We have come to the humbling conclusion that knowledge is forever evolving, that while we have reached certain plateaus of erudition, we can rest on none of them. They serve as new launching pads for our next scientific endeavor. Scientific method—a pillar of the foundation of our modern civilization—is built from a value system, and these values are themselves constantly under scrutiny and modulated as our needs and sophistication evolve.

History shares many of these same epistemological values, and restraints, with science. Although there is no opportunity for experimentation and the "What if . . . " question can only be rhetorical in determining historical facts, historians, as public agents of our collective past, are committed to proceeding by objective means to recover our antecedents. While there is potentially wide latitude in interpretation, clearly historical narratives should be veridical, which is determined not by some measure against nature as in science, but in the ongoing forum of criticism and debate. Therefore we have many histories, because no single narrative, chronicle, movie, testimony, museum, or archive is complete. No single historian, or even school of historical analyses, can hope to depict anything but a small aspect of the past. Each perspective is different and precious. We need many reports, which even in their collected whole can never truly capture that past. But we must try, and this is the other dimension in which history shares close affinity with memory: History becomes moral in the public domain just as memory is a moral activity for the individual.

We regard the past through the prism of our current values, and we bring the past into the present—and even project it into the future as our "manifest destiny." We reinterpret our social evolution from the vantage of our current understanding, and although historians are wary of presentism—that prejudice of seeing the past in terms of our own cultural moment—we nevertheless cannot totally escape the strictures of our imbibed culture with all the attendant orientation it bestows. In the acts of shared memory (and forgetting), a historical character emerges, and thus history, when viewed as a social activity, becomes a critical means by which we define ourselves as a group, analogous with the way in which memory helps define the individual. Memory is constitutive of our personal identities, and history, being firmly situated in the civic domain, becomes constituent of social identity. As the historian Paula Fredriksen cogently puts it: "[T]he past is not . . . preserved so much as remade in the image of the present: The past is too important to be allowed to exist. . . . [The] narrative can reveal . . . only the retrospective moment, and the retrospective self." In that act, our collective identity is forged.

I am caught on this swing between history and memory, between a narrative of collective experience and an intimate recollection. My memory becomes public as I recall the past here, and I do so not as formal history (and I make no apology for any laxity in this recording), but as an attempt to capture my past and bring it into our present for public scrutiny. Through confession I have hoped to articulate experience that reflects our common moral quandary and speculate how I, as an individual, might articulate a communal problem with a public voice. As we reflect on the triumph of scientific medicine and its technological imperative we are reminded of a more ancient calling, one that both history and memory must serve us to reconstruct and orient us in the care of another. As I've become aware of my part in the historical record of late twentieth-century medicine, I have sought expression of that calling in the echo of my distant experience. Only by exploring the caves of my memory can I begin to fashion a response to our current predicament, for the past, no matter how elusive, remains our anchor; to lose that tether is to be set hopelessly adrift.

Bibliographic Notes

Those interested in obtaining references to issues raised in this essay are either referred to my previous writings or pushed gently in the direction to those works that have particularly provoked my own thinking. I make no effort here at offering a comprehensive bibliographic survey, but must be satisfied with providing the reader with a few suggestions. Those texts alluded to but not directly quoted from are listed here. At the end of these general referrals, I have included the specific citations of quoted material.

Regarding medical education, see my article, "The Two Faces of Medical Education: Flexner and Osler Revisited." (*Journal of the Royal Society of Medicine* 85 [1992]: 598–602). There one will find references documenting the historical development of modern clinical training, the role of Osler and Peabody, and discussion of the current fledgling efforts to teach medical humanities. Those more interested in exploring the lives and influence of Osler and Peabody should read the classic study of Harvey Cushing, *The Life of Sir William Osler* (Oxford, Clarendon Press, 1925), or the recent shorter study by Charles S. Bryan, *Osler: Inspirations from a Great Physician* (Oxford: Oxford University Press, 1997); and *The Caring Physician: The Life of Dr. Francis W. Peabody* by Paul Oglesby (Boston: The Countway Library, 1991). The relationship of basic science to medical education and practice is a rich subject, and I would suggest for more comprehensive treatment *The Structure of American Medical Practice, 1875–1941* by George Rosen (Philadelphia: University of Pennsylvania Press, 1983); *American Medicine in Transition, 1840–1910* by John S. Haller (Urbana: University of Illinois Press, 1981); *Learning to Heal: The Development of American Medical Education* by Kenneth M. Ludmerer (New York: Basic Books, 1985); *American Medical Schools and the Prac-*

tice of Medicine: A History by William G. Rothstein (Oxford: Oxford University Press, 1987); and *The Care of Strangers: The Rise of America's Hospital System* (New York: Basic Books, 1987). John Harley Warren gives an excellent summary of changing perspectives on science in medicine in "Science in Medicine," *Osiris*, 2d series, 1 (1985):37–58.

Our current scientific orientation in medicine is discussed in my article, "Darwinian Aftershocks: Repercussions in Late Twentieth-Century Medicine" (*Journal of the Royal Society of Medicine* 87 [1994]: 27–31), and for a full discussion of the reductionist revolution in biology at the end of the nineteenth century, see my study of early immunology, co-authored with Leon Chernyak: *Metchnikoff and the Origins of Immunology: From Metaphor to Theory* (New York: Oxford University Press, 1991). For the perspective of science responding to the opportunity of support from medicine, see *From Medical Chemistry to Biochemistry: The Making of a Biomedical Discipline* by Robert E. Kohler (Cambridge: Cambridge University Press, 1982).

For me, the most influential text regarding the development of twentieth-century medicine as a social institution and the economic consequences of the triumph of medical doctors over other kinds of clinical practitioners is Paul Starr's *The Social Transformation of American Medicine: The Rise of a Sovereign Profession and the Making of a Vast Industry* (New York: Basic Books, 1982). With the explosion of critiques of contemporary medical practice and the economic consequences, I am hard pressed to choose between the various ideologues. Suffice it to note that the onslaught may conveniently (if not arbitrarily) be assigned to Ivan Illich's *The Medical Nemesis: The Expropriation of Health* (New York: Random House, 1976), a product of the radical 1960s, but still relevant today in tracing the erosion of public trust in the physician. Of those who were most adamant in their criticism of physicians serving as society's gatekeepers, see Thomas Szasz's *The Myth of Mental Illness* (New York: Hoeber-Harper, 1961), which specifically attacks the institutionalization of the mentally ill, but was also seen as a strike against the authoritarian posture assumed by a paternalistic medicine more generally.

Recent analyses of the economics and politics of health care have appeared in droves, and I mention only a few of the more interesting studies: George Anders, *Health Against Wealth: HMOs and the Breakdown of Medical Trust* (New York: Houghton Mifflin, 1996); Robert H. Blank, *The Price of Life: The Future of American Health Care* (New York: Columbia University Press, 1997); Regina E. Herzlinger, *Market-Driven Health Care: Who Wins, Who Loses in the Transformation of America's Largest Service Industry* (Reading, MA: Addison-Wesley, 1997); and David J. Rothman, *Beginnings Count: The Technological Imperative in American Health Care* (New York: Oxford University Press, 1997). An accessible summary of the current efforts to assess quality of care appeared as a series of six articles in *The New England Journal of Medicine* 335 (September 19–October 24, 1996).

Regarding philosophical matters, there are several general topics that have dominated this essay. The first concerns current moral philosophy, and here I would simply refer one to the writings of John Caputo, Alasdair MacIntyre, and Bernard Williams for excellent expositions of general contemporary ethics in the Anglo-American tradition. Representative texts include John Caputo, *Against Ethics* (Bloomington: Indiana University Press, 1993); note an interesting critique of Levinas. Alasdair MacIntyre, *After Virtue,* 2d ed. (Notre Dame: Notre Dame University Press, 1984); see especially chapter 15 for an articulate statement of how "narrative" is fundamentally moral, the "essential genre for the characterization of human actions" (p. 208). Bernard Williams, *Ethics and the Limits of Philosophy* (Cambridge: Harvard University Press, 1985.) The more basic argument concerns the very possibility of doing philosophy, and here the writings of Ludwig Wittgenstein have been most influential. For an accessible introduction to his thought see Alan Janik and Stephen Toulmin, *Wittgenstein's Vienna* (New York: Touchstone, 1973), and for more sophisticated philosophical comment, Joachim Schulte, *Wittgenstein: An Introduction* (Albany: State University of New York Press, 1992); William H. Bartley, III, *Wittgenstein,* 2d ed. (LaSalle, IL: Open Court, 1985); and Judith Genova, *Wittgenstein: A Way of Seeing* (New York: Routledge, 1995). For a particularly accessible study of how Wittgenstein approached ethics see Russell Nieli, *Wittgenstein: From Mysticism to Ordinary Language* (Albany: State University of New York Press, 1987). Those interested in the unstable state of contemporary philosophy more generally should see John Rajchman and Cornel West (eds.), *Postanalytic Philosophy* (New York: Columbia University Press, 1985); Kenneth Baynes,

James Bohman, and Thomas McCarthy (eds.), *After Philosophy: End or Transformation?* (Cambridge, MA: MIT Press, 1986); and James Ogilvy (ed.), *Revisioning Philosophy* (Albany, NY: State University of New York Press, 1992).

Medical ethics is a complicated terrain to traverse, and I would suggest both specific and general treatments. H. Tristram Engelhardt, Jr., *The Foundations of Bioethics* (New York: Oxford University Press) is an excellent sustained philosophical argument, which has been influential in these circles. There are two editions of the text; the first (published in 1986) is firmly committed to the ideal of autonomy, whereas the second edition (1996) has muted that point of view for one embracing a softer communalism. The transition in itself is quite important. Another interesting approach using communal moral philosophy is an application of Josiah Royce's "loyalty ethics" by Griffin Trotter *(The Loyal Physician: Roycean Ethics and the Practice of Medicine.* Nashville: Vanderbilt University Press, 1997), whose argument is similar in important respects to MacIntyre's *After Virtue* (op. cit.). Trotter maintains that the physician, in reconciling his or her own needs for self-differentiation with communitarian needs, must adopt the ideal of loyalty, conceived (in what some might regard as naive idealism) as "the willing, thoroughgoing, and practical devotion to a cause" (p. 9). That cause, expressed in the individual doctor-patient encounter, only takes its full meaning, and stability, in the context of the greater medical community, of which the entire health care industry, patients, and would-be patients (all of us) aspire to optimal community health. Thus virtue ethics, loyalty being the unifying virtue, intertwines the notion of selfhood with the notion of community. The quixotically disinclined might regard all of this as a fancy way of saying that a physician should be dedicated to the ideals of medicine, but if one seeks serious discussion of why "we will suppose, for a while, that a moral life is something grand" (p. 2), then this book is worth examining.

Of those books offering a more eclectic philosophical overview, perhaps the best is Tom L. Beauchamp and James F. Childress, *Principles of Biomedical Ethics,* 4th ed., (New York Oxford University Press, 1994). Other influential texts include Robert Veatch, *A Theory of Medical Ethics* (New York: Basic Books, 1981), and Edmund D. Pellegrino and David C. Thomasma, *A Philosophical Basis of Medical Practice* (New York: Oxford University Press, 1981). Also consider *Underpinnings of Medical Ethics,* by Edmond A. Murphy, James J. Buzow, and Edward L. Suarez-Murias (Baltimore: The Johns Hopkins University Press, 1997), a text which reflects the senior author's penchant for logic and systematic thinking; and the classic text dealing with the philosophical standing of the patient, Paul Ramsey's *The Patient as Person: Explorations in Medical Ethics* (New Haven: Yale University Press, 1970). The theological basis of medical ethics may be surveyed in *On Moral Medicine: Theological Perspectives in Medical Ethics,* eds. Stephen E. Lammers and Allen Verhey (Grand Rapids, MI: Eerdmans Publishing Company, 1987).

For more practical treatments, consider Terrance F. Ackerman and Carson Strong, *A Casebook of Medical Ethics* (New York: Oxford University Press, 1989) and John C. Fletcher, Norman Quist, and Albert R. Jonsen, eds., *Ethics Consultation in Health Care* (Ann Arbor, MI: Health Administration Press, 1989). A concise but comprehensive compendium and explanation of patients' rights is offered by George J. Annas, *The Rights of Patients: The Basic ACLU Guide to Patient Rights,* 2d ed. (Carbondale: Southern Illinois University Press, 1989); recent study of patient autonomy in the clinical setting is given by Jan C. Hofmann, Neil S. Wenger, Roger B. Davis, et al., "Patient preferences for communication with physicians about end-of-life decisions," *Annals of Internal Medicine* 127 (1997): 1–12; for judicial comment concerning physician fiduciary responsibility, see Marc A. Rodwin, "Strains in the fiduciary metaphor: Divided physician loyalties and the obligations in a changing health care system," *American Journal of Law and Medicine* 21 (1995): 241–257. A portrait of real life medical ethics in action is well provided by Robert Zussman, *Intensive Care: Medical Ethics and the Medical Profession* (Chicago: The University of Chicago Press, 1992).

Excellent histories of medical ethics are offered by David J. Rothman's *Strangers at the Bedside: A History of How Law and Bioethics Transformed Medical Decision Making* (New York: Basic Books, 1991) and Albert R. Jonsen's *The Birth of Bioethics* (New York: Oxford University Press, 1998). A more concise history is presented by Robert Baker, "The History of Medical Ethics," in *Companion Encyclopedia of the History of Medicine,* eds. W. F. Bynum and R. Porter (New York and London: Routledge, 1993), pp. 852–887. To taste the postmodern influence in medical ethics, see Paul A. Komesaroff, ed., *Troubled Bodies. Critical Perspectives on Postmodernism, Medical Ethics, and the Body* (Durham: Duke University Press, 1995). For positions generally affiliated with my own views on applied ethics, one might sample Seymour M. Glick, "Humanistic medicine in a modern age," *New England Journal of Medicine* 304 (1981): 1036–1038, and David Roochnik, "Applied ethics: Some Platonic questions," *Philosophy in Context* 17 (1987): 40–51.

Recent writing in medical philosophy more generally is surprisingly sparse. The most important are translated European works: Georges Canguilhem, *The Normal and the Pathological* (New York: ZONE Books, 1989); Michel Foucault, *The Birth of the Clinic: An Archaeology of Medical Perception* (New York: Random House, 1973); and Hans-Georg Gadamer, *The Enigma of Health* (Palo Alto: Stanford, 1996). Two accessible overviews are Edmund D. Pellegrino and David C. Thomasma, *A Philosophical Basis of Medical Practice* (op. cit.) and Henrik R. Wulff, Stig Pedersen, and Raben Rosenberg, *Philosophy of Medicine: An Introduction,* 2d ed. (Oxford: Blackwell Scientific Publications, 1990). The position of medical philosophy relative to its offspring, medical ethics, is readily appreciated given the few titles available that deal with the broadest questions philosophy might address in medicine compared to the libraries of comment concerning medical ethics.

In America, it seems that we have chosen to teach humanistic medicine sociologically: A discipline has emerged that treats the philosophical issues by attempting to define various comparative cultural perspectives of the experience of illness, tracing the influence of social factors on health and disease, and delineating the "culture" of medicine and medical practice. These are ostensibly sociological or anthropological analyses, but one might easily discern many of what I have regarded as philosophical questions disguised in these discussions. A good introduction to this approach is offered in Gail E. Henderson, Nancy M. P. King, Ronald P. Strauss, Sue E. Estroff, and Larry R. Churchill, eds., *The Social Medicine Reader* (Durham: Duke University Press, 1997) and Uta Gerhardt, *Ideas about Illness: An Intellectual and Political History of Medical Sociology* (New York: New York University Press, 1989).

As to the general topic of selfhood, Charles Taylor's *The Sources of the Self: The Making of Modern Identity* (Cambridge: Harvard University

Press, 1989) is the best overview, and for a more detailed treatment of my own views, see my book, *The Immune Self: Theory or Metaphor?* (New York: Cambridge University Press, 1994). A more complete discussion of Nietzsche may be found there, and also in my "A typology of Nietzsche's biology" *(Biology and Philosophy* 9 [1994]: 24–44). Regarding Nietzsche's concept of health and illness, see my article coauthored with Scott H. Podolsky, "Nietzsche's conception of health—the idealization of struggle," in *Nietzsche, Epistemology, and Philosophy of Science. Nietzsche and the Sciences*, vol. 2, Babette Babich and Robert S. Cohen (eds.), (Dordrecht: Kluwer Academic Publishers, 1998, pp. 338–353). My views of Nietzsche's ethics is detailed in two papers: "On the transvaluation of values: Nietzsche contra Foucault," in *Science, Mind and Art: Papers in Honor of Robert S. Cohen,* Kostas Gavroglu, John Stachel, and Marx W. Wartofsky (eds.), (Dordrecht: Kluwer Academic Publishers, 1995. pp. 349–367); and "From the self to the other: Building a philosophy of medicine," in *Meta-Medical Ethics: The Philosophical Foundations of Bioethics,* Michael A. Grodin (ed.) (Dordrecht: Kluwer Academic Publishers, 1995. pp. 149–195). There is a huge library of Nietzsche studies, and I would single out two for their treatment of themes discussed here. First, concerning the self, I recommend Leslie P. Thiele's *Friedrich Nietzsche and the Politics of the Soul* (Princeton: Princeton University Press, 1990), and for a more detailed analysis of the eternal recurrence from the perspective adopted here see Arthur Nehamas, *Nietzsche: Life as Literature* (Cambridge: Harvard University Press, 1985).

My interpretation of Levinas's philosophy is detailed in two papers: "From the self to the other," op. cit., and "Outside the subject: Levinas's Jewish perspective on time" (*Graduate Faculty Philosophy Journal* Fall, 1998). Levinas's major works have been translated, the most important being *Totality and Infinity* [1961], (Pittsburgh: Duquesne University Press, 1969) and *Otherwise than Being or Beyond Essence* [1974], (Dordrecht: Kluwer Academic Publishers, 1991). Excellent general reviews of his work include Edith Wyschogrod's *Emmanuel Levinas: The Problem of Ethical Metaphysics* (The Hague: Martinus Nijhoff, 1974) and Arthur Peperzak, *To the Other: An Introduction to the Philosophy of Emmanuel Levinas* (Purdue: Purdue University Press, 1993). Valuable essays are contained in Robert Bernasconi and Simon Critchley (eds.), *Rereading Levinas*

(Bloomington: Indiana University Press, 1991) and R. A. Cohen, (ed.), *Face to Face with Levinas* (Albany: State University of New York Press, 1986). A closely aligned philosophical position orginating from a different tradition is given by Knud E. Logstrup, *The Ethical Demand* (Philadelphia: Fortress Press, 1971), and for a more "sociological" rendition of how ethics is aporetic and nonfoundational, see Zygmunt Bauman, *Postmodern Ethics*, (Oxford: Blackwell Publishers, 1993). The relational philosophy I have espoused here also comes under a different philosophical title of *dependency*; see Richard Vance's "Medicine as a dependent tradition: Historical and ethical reflections," *Perspectives in Biology and Medicine* 28 (1985): 282–302.

Writings on illness, suffering and death have found much general interest. This genre achieved its place among best-selling titles with Elisabeth Kubler-Ross's *On Death and Dying* (New York: Macmillan, 1969); more recently, Sherwin Nuland's *How We Die: Reflections on Life's Final Chapter* (New York: Knopf, 1993) achieved popular and critical acclaim and truly is a poignant witnessing statement. Personal accounts of dying, like Peter Noll's *In the Face of Death* (New York: Penguin, 1989), and of recovery, such as Norman Cousins's *Anatomy of an Illness as Perceived by the Patient* (New York: Norton, 1979), or May Sarton's *After the Stroke: A Journal* (New York: Norton, 1988), are often inspiring testaments that complement more analytical studies. Of the latter, Eric Cassell, *The Nature of Suffering and the Goals of Medicine* (New York: Oxford University Press, 1991); S. Kay Toombs, *The Meaning of Illness* (Dordrecht: Kluwer Academic Publishers, 1992); and Anne Hunsaker Hawkins, *Reconstructing Illness: Studies in Pathography* (Purdue: Purdue University Press, 1993) are representative of scholarship in this area.

The more specific problem of physician empathy toward the patient has also become an academic area of scholarship, and three anthologies offering diverse perspectives are John D. Stoeckle (ed.), *Encounters between Patients and Doctors* (Cambridge: The MIT Press, 1987); Howard M. Spiro, Mary G. M. Curnen, Enid Peschel, and Deborah St. James (eds.), *Empathy and the Practice of Medicine: Beyond Pills and the Scapel* (New Haven: Yale University Press, 1993), and Ellen Singer More and Maureen A. Milligan (eds.), *The Empathetic Practitioner* (Rutgers: Rutgers University Press, 1994). I have deliberately not delved into the more complex arena of why empathy is a problem, that is, the possible psychological forms of resistance doctors experience in their care of patients. An informative introduction to this question is Howard F. Stein, (ed.), *The Psychodynamics of Medical Practice: Unconscious Factors in Patient Care* (Berkeley: University of California Press, 1985).

Finally, the central role of narrative, serving both to illustrate the dynamics of professional compassion and the resulting moral position developed here, is explored from a different perspective in Kathryn Montgomery Hunter, *Doctors' Stories: The Narrative Structure of Medical Knowledge* (Princeton: Princeton University Press, 1991) and more generally in Alasdair MacIntyre's, *After Virtue* (op. cit.). Critiques of this orientation may be found in Hilde L. Nelson, *Stories and Their Limitations* (New York and London: Routledge, 1997). But perhaps the best descriptions of the empathetic doctor-patient encounter are those literary portraits of the compassionate physician, of which John Berger, *A Fortunate Man: The Story of a Country Doctor* (New York: Vintage [1967] 1997) is among the best.

References

Complete bibliographic citations to quoted material are listed below by chapter.

Introduction: Alasdair MacIntyre, *After Virtue*, 2d ed., op. cit. p. 216; Statistics are taken from Andrew Hacker, "The medicine in our future," *New York Review of Books* 44 (1997): 26–31.

Chapter 1: Francis W. Peabody, "The physician and the laboratory," *Boston Medical and Surgical Journal* 187 (1922): 324–327; idem., *The Care of the Patient* (Cambridge: Harvard University Press, 1927), pp. 10, 48

Chapter 2: Susan Sontag, *Illness and Its Metaphors and AIDS and Its Metaphors* (New York: Farrar, Straus & Giroux, 1989), pp. 43–44; Max Navarre, "Fighting the victim label," in *AIDS: Cultural Analysis, Cultural Activisim,* Douglas Crimp (ed.) (Cambridge: The MIT Press, 1988), pp. 143–146.

Chapter 3: William James, *The Principles of Psychology* (Cambridge: Harvard University Press, 1983), p. 290; C. S. Lewis, "Preface," in *The Hierarchy of Heaven and Earth* by D. E. Harding (New York: Harper and Brothers, 1952), p. 10.

Chapter 4:   Zygmunt Bauman, *Postmodern Ethics*, Oxford: Blackwell Publishers, 1993, p. 13; John Caputo, *Against Ethics*, op. cit. p. 7; Bernard Williams, *Ethics and the Limits of Philosophy*, op. cit., pp. 4, 8; Aladair MacIntyre, *After Virtue*, op. cit., p. 2; William James, *The Principles of Psychology*, op. cit., p. 278; Norman Daniels, *Justice and Justification: Reflective Equilibrium in Theory and Practice* (New York: Cambridge University Press, 1996); L. Wayne Sumner and Joseph Boyle, "Introduction," in *Philosophical Perspectives on Bioethics*, eds. L. Wayne Sumner and Joseph Boyle (Toronto: University of Toronto Press, 1996), p. 5; Maimonides quoted by Shimon M. Glick, "Research in a Hierarchy of Values," *The Mount Sinai Journal of Medicine* 59 (1992): 102–107; *idem.*, "The empathetic physician: Nature and nurture," in *Empathy and the Practice of Medicine: Beyond Pills and the Scapel*, eds. H. M. Spiro, M. G. M. Curnen, E. Peschel, and D. St. James, op. cit., pp. 85–102. (quotation from p. 90).

Chapter 5:   Howard Brody, *Ethical Decisions in Medicine*, 2d ed. (Boston: Little, Brown, and Co., 1981), p. 5; C. S. Lewis, *The Abolition of Man*, New York: Macmillan, 1947, p. 40; Marc A. Rodwin, "Strains in the fiduciary metaphor" op. cit., pp. 249, 254; Savonarola quoted in Maurcie B. Strauss (ed.), *Familiar Medical Quotations* (Boston: Little, Brown & Co., 1968), p. 399; Nathaniel Hawthorne, *The Scarlet Letter* (New York: Dell Publishing Co., 1960), pp. 158–159 (Chapter 9); John Berger, *A Country Doctor* (op. cit.) quotes from, in order, pp. 75, 76, and 62.

Chapter 6:   Milan Kundera, *The Unbearable Lightness of Being* (New York: Harper and Row, 1987), p. 5.

Epilogue: Paula Fredriksen, "Paul and Augustine: conversion narratives, orthodox traditions, and the retrospective self," *Journal of Theological Studies* 37 (1986): 33–34.

Index

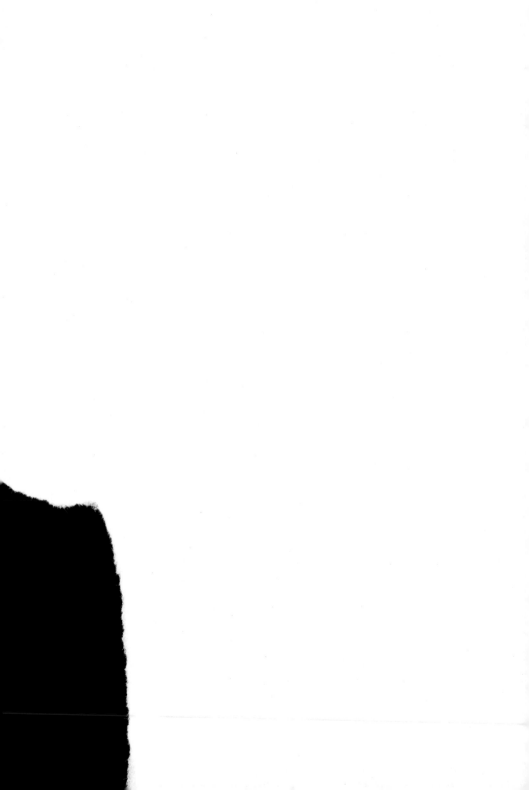

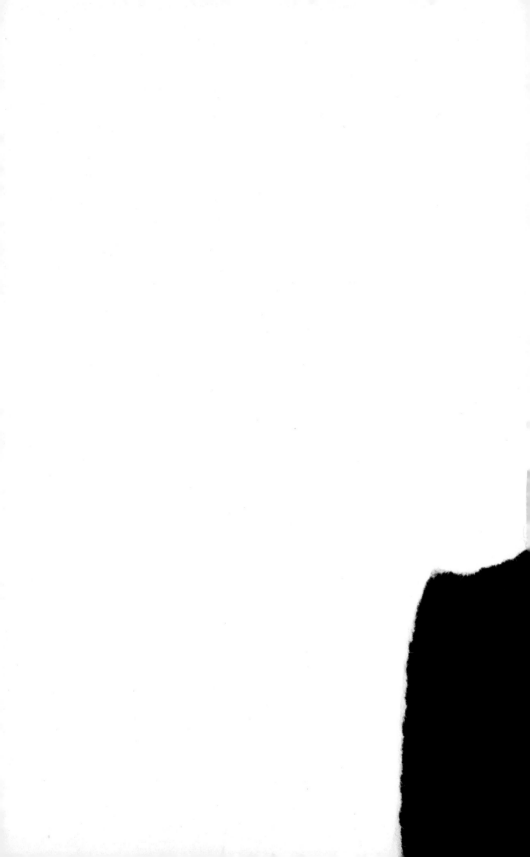